HUMANISTIC NURSING

Josephine G. Paterson, DNSc, RN
Loretta T. Zderad, PhD, RN

Pub. No. 41 – 2218

 National League for Nursing · New York

17819495

This is a rerelease of a volume originally published in 1976.

Manufactured in the United States of America

PREFACE

Somewhere there's a child a crying
Somewhere there's a child a crying
Somewhere there's a child a crying
Crying for freedom in South Africa.[1]

But until someone hears the cry and responds, the child will continue to suffer the oppression of the current South African regime; and the world will continue to be less than it could be. To cry aloud when there seems no chance of being heard, belies a hope—perhaps an inherently human trait—that someone, somewhere, somehow will hear that cry and respond to it.

This same hope, that someone would hear and respond, allowed existential psychologist Viktor Frankl to survive the systematic torture and degradation in Nazi death camps. As Frankl and others sought their way, they found meaning and salvation "through love and in love;" and by choosing to believe that "life still waited for him, that a human being waited for his return."[2]

There is power in the call of one person and the potential response of another; and incredible power when the potential response becomes real. There is the power for each person to change as she becomes more than she was before the dialogue. There is the power to transcend the situation as two people engage the events that are whirling around them and together try to make sense of their worlds and find a meaning to their existence. When the call and response between two people is as honest as it can be, there is the revolutionary power which the poet Muriel Rukeyser speaks of:

What would happen if one woman told the truth about her life?
The world would split open.[3]

---

[1] *Azanian Freedom Song.* Lyrics by Otis Williams, music by Bernice Johnson Reagon. Washington, DC: Songtalk Publishing Co., 1982
[2] Frankl, Viktor. *Man's Search For Meaning.* Boston: Beacon Press, 1959
[3] Rukeyser, Muriel. "Kathe Kollwitz," in *By a Woman Writ,* ed. Joan Goulianos. New York : Bobbs Merrill, 1973, p. 374.

The call and response of an authentic dialogue between a nurse and patient has great power—the power to change the lived experiences of both patient and nurse, to change the situation, to change the world. It is the same authenticity we search for in relationships with our friends and lovers. The person who really listens to what we are saying, who really tries to understand our lived experiences of the world and who asks the same from us. When found, it brings the same exhilirating feeling of self-affirmation and the comforting feeling of well-being.

For, if as holistic beings we are the implicate order explicating itself, as suggested by Bohm[4] and Newman[5] among others, then the responsibilities of those who would help (e.g., nurses) include making sense out of the chaos that can occur as illness disrupts past order and as the ever-present threat of non-being disrupts all order. When we are successful in helping patients and their loved ones make sense of their lives by bringing meaning to them, we make sense of and bring meaning to our own.

And when we help create meaning, it is easier to remember why we chose nursing and why we continue to choose it despite what an underpaid and undervalued job it has become in today's marketplace. These are the moments when by a look or a word or a touch, the patient lets us know that he understands what is happening to him, what his choices are, and what he is going to do; that he knows we know; and that each knows that the other knows. When we get past our science and theories, our technical prowess, our titles and positions of influence, it is this shared moment of authenticity— between patient and nurse—that makes us smile and allows us to move forward in our own life projects.

Nurse educators who seek such authentic exchanges with their students enjoy similar moments. The same can be said of deans of schools of nursing, administrators of delivery systems, executives and staff of nursing and professional organizations, and colleagues on a research project. It is the authentic dialogue between people that makes any activity worthwhile regardless of whether or not it is called successful by others.

When Josephine G. Paterson and Loretta T. Zderad first published their book *Humanistic Nursing* in 1976, society was in the midst of the new women's movement and nurses were going through the phase of assertiveness training, dressing for success, and learning to play the games that mother never taught us. Since then, nurses have moved into many sectors of society and have held power as we have never held it before. We have proved ourselves as politicians, administrators, researchers, and writers. We have refined our abilities to assess, diagnose, treat, and evalute. We've raised money and balanced budgets. We've networked, organized, and formed coalitions.

Yet, individually we are uneasy and collectively we are unable to articulate a vision clear enough so that others will join us. This re-issue of Paterson and

[4] Bohm, David. *Wholeness and the Implicate Order.* London: Ark, 1980.
[5] Newman, Margaret. *Health As Expanding Consciousness.* St. Louis: C.V. Mosby Company, 1986.

Zderad's classic work will help to remind us of another way of developing our power. Perhaps we can, once again, look for and call for authentic dialogue with our patients, our students, and our colleagues. Paterson and Zderad are clear in their method: discuss, question, convey, clarify, argue, and reflect. They remind us of our uniqueness and our commonality. They tell us that it is necessary to do with and be with each other in order for any one of us to grow. They help us celebrate the power of our choices.

Is it ironic and fortunate that *Humanistic Nursing* should be re-issued now when it is needed even more than it was during the late 1970s? Then, humanitarianism was in vogue. Now, it is under attack as a secular religion.

Today, the technocratic imperative infiltrates an ever-increasing number of our lived experiences; and it becomes more difficult to ignore or dismiss Habermas's analysis that all interests have become technical rather than human.[6] As health care becomes increasingly commercial the profound experiences of living and dying are discussed in terms of profit and loss. Life itself is the focus of public debates about whether surrogacy involves a whole baby being bought and sold or only half of a baby, since one half already "belongs" to the natural father and so he cannot buy what he already owns.

We have many choices before us: to adopt the values of commerce and redesign health care systems accordingly; to accept competition as the modus operandi or insist on other measures for people in need; to decide who will be cared for, who won't, who will pay, and how much?

Perhaps it is time for us to turn away from the exchange between buyers and sellers, providers and consumers; and turn back to an exchange between two people trying to understand the space they share. Perhaps it is time for a shared dialogue with patients for whom the questions are most vital? Perhaps we need to hear their call and respond authentically. Perhaps they need to hear ours? For only then, as Paterson and Zderad have made quite clear, will our lived experiences in health care have any real meaning.

Patricia Moccia PhD, RN
Associate Professor and Chair
Department of Nursing Education
Teachers College Columbia University

---

[6] Habermas, Jurgen. *Knowledge and Human Interest.* (trans. J. Shapiro.) Boston: Beacon Press, 1971

CONTENTS

THEORETICAL ROOTS

1
HUMANISTIC NURSING PRACTICE THEORY

Substantively this chapter introduces two aspects of the humanistic nursing practice theory: first, what this theory proposes and, second, how the proposals of the theory evolved.

Concisely, humanistic nursing practice theory proposes that nurses consciously and deliberately approach nursing as an existential experience. Then, they reflect on the experience and phenomenologically describe the calls they receive, their responses, and what they come to know from their presence in the nursing situation. It is believed that compilation and complementary syntheses of these phenomenological descriptions over time will build and make explicit a science of nursing.

HUMANISTIC NURSING: ITS MEANING

Nursing is an experience lived between human beings. Each nursing situation reciprocally evokes and affects the expression and manifestations of these human beings' capacity for and condition of existence. In a nurse this implies a responsibility for the condition of herself or being. The term "humanistic nursing" was selected thoughtfully to designate this theoretical pursuit to reaffirm and floodlight this responsible characteristic as fundamentally inherent to all artful-scientific nursing. Humanistic nursing embraces more than a benevolent technically competent subject–object one-way relationship guided by a nurse in behalf of another. Rather it dictates that nursing is a responsible searching, transactional relationship whose meaningfulness demands conceptualization founded on a nurse's existential awareness of self and of the other.

3

EXISTENTIAL EXPERIENCE

Uniqueness–Otherness

Existential experience infers human awareness of the self and of otherness. It calls for a recognition of each man as existing singularly in-his-situation and struggling and striving with his fellows for survival and becoming, for confirmation of his existence and understanding of its meaning.

Martin Buber, philosophical anthropologist and rabbi, expressed artfully this uniqueness, struggle, and potential of each man. He said:

> "Sent forth from the natural domain of species into the hazard of the solitary category, [man] surrounded by the air of a chaos which came into being with him, secretly and bashfully he watches for a Yes which allows him to be and which can come to him only from one human person to another."[1]

With such uniqueness of each human being as a given, an assumed fact, only each person can describe or choose the evolvement of the project which is himself-in-his situation. This awesome and lonely human capacity for choice and novel evolvement presents both hope and fear as regards the unfolding of human "moreness." Uniqueness is a universal capacity of the human species. So, "all-at-once," while each man is unique; paradoxically, he is also like his fellows. His very uniqueness is a characteristic of his commonality with all other men.

Authenticity–Experiencing

In humanistic nursing existential awareness calls for an authenticity with one's self. As a visionary aim, such authenticity, self-in-touchness, is more than what usually is termed intellectual awareness. Auditory, olfactory, oral, visual, tactile, kinesthetic, and visceral responses are involved and each can convey unique meaning to man's consciousness. In-touchness with these sensations and our responses informs us about our quality of being, our thereness, our degree of presence with others. The kind of "between" we live with others depends on both our degree of awareness and the meaning we attribute to this awareness. This awareness, reflected on, sometimes shared with a responsible other for reality testing, offers us opportunity for broadening our meaning base, for becoming more—more in accord with our potential for humanness.

Perhaps a statement made by Dr. Gene Phillips, professor of education at Boston University, will clarify the importance I attach to each nurse becoming as much as she can be. He said, "The more mature we are the less it is necessary for us to exclude." Presently I would paraphrase this statement

---

[1] Martin Buber, "Distance and Relation," trans. Ronald Gregor Smith, in *The Knowledge of Man,* ed. Maurice Friedman (New York: Harper & Row, Publishers, 1965), p. 71.

and say, the more of ourselves we do not have to exclude, the more of the other we can be open to. Our self-awareness, in-touchness, self-acceptance, actualization of our potential allows us to share with others so they can become in relationship with us.

In this kind of existential relating, presence with another, a nurse is confronted with man as singular in his own peculiar angular, biased, or shaded reality. It becomes apparent that each has his very own lived world. So one might describe human existence as man–world as some refer to man as mind–body, using a hyphen rather than "and." Man's universal species commonality and peculiar perplexing noncommonality, has this manness, affect and constantly interplay with one another. This arena of interplay is complicated further by man's capacity for nondeterminedness, his ability for envisioning and considering a variety of alternatives and choosing selectively. Often these alternatives are experienced as contradictory and inconsistent. Humanistic nursing calls forth in the nurse the struggle of recognizing the complexity of men's relating in the nursing world as "just how man is" and his nature, his human condition, as searching, experiencing, and an unfolding becoming.

Moreness–Choice

How can a nurse let herself know her human responses and the breadth and depth of the possibilities called forth by the other? How can she be, search, experience, become in an accord with the calls and responses of her lived nursing world? It is a chosen, deliberate life-long process. The process itself is generative. One experience opens the door for the next. In humanistic nursing practice theory we call this kind of experiencing authentic, genuine, or "letting be what is." It is man conscious of himself, not necessarily acting out, but aware of his human responses to his world and their meanings to him. This quality of personal authenticity allows one's responsible chosen actions to be based in human knowledge rather than human defensiveness. Man is a knowing place. From education and living experience one assumes an initial innate force in human beingness that moves man to come to know his own and others' angular views of the world. Humanistic nursing is concerned with these angular views, these differences being viewed by nurses responsibly and as realities that are beyond the negative–positive, good–evil standard of judgement. Or, for example, nursing is concerned with how this particular man, with his particular history, experiences being labeled with this general diagnosis and being admitted, discharged, and living out his life with his condition as he views it in-his-world.

Man has the inherent capacity to respond to other man as other man. Only each unique nurse faced with the chaos of her alternatives in a situation can then choose either to relate or not to relate and how to relate in-her-nursing-world to others. Choosing to and how to relate or respond cannot be superimposed on man from the outside by another. A person, to a degree, can be coerced to behave outwardly in a certain way. For example, physically, in a spatial sense, a nurse can be ordered into parallel existence with another. Being existentially and genuinely present with another is different. This human mode of being is chosen and controlled by the self. It takes responsible self-ordering that can arise only in the spirit of one's own disciplined being.

Value–Nonvalue

To offer genuine presence to others, a belief must exist within a person that such presence is of value and makes a difference in a situation. If it is a value for a nurse, it will be offered in her nursing situation. Libraries, concrete buildings bursting with words of great thinkers, support the value of genuine presence and authentic dialogue between persons. Consider the literary works that have conveyed or reflected this message throughout the existence of intellectual man. Plato, Rousseau, Goethe, Proust, Nietzsche, Whitehead, Jung, May, Frankl, Hesse, de Chardin, Bergson, Marcel and Buber effortlessly come to mind.

Many nurses are genuine presences in the nursing situation. Some have tried to share their experiences; some have not. And, there are those who are not genuine presences in the nursing situation. One wonders if this has influenced the distinctions nurses have made over the years with certainty when considering their nurse contemporaries. Often one hears, "she is a good nurse, a natural." These positive critics are often up against it when asked, "why, how, what?" Descriptive literary conceptualizations of nursing that reflect this quality of nurse-being (presence, intersubjectiveness) call for nurses willing to search out and bring to awareness, the mysteries of their commonplace, their familiar, and to appreciate the unique ideas, values, and meanings fundamental to their practice. Conceptualization of these qualities by practicing nurses is basic and necessary to the development of a science and an actualized profession of nursing.

PHENOMENOLOGICAL DESCRIPTION

Phenomenology directs us to the study of the "thing itself." The existential literature, descriptions of what man has come to know and understand in his experience, has evolved from the use of the phenomenological approach. In the humanistic nursing practice theory the "thing itself" is the existentially experienced nursing situation. Both phenomenology and existentialism value experience, man's capacities for surprise and knowing, and honor the evolving of the "new."

What Does Humanistic Nursing Practice
Theory Ask the Nurse to Describe?

Nurses experience with other human beings peak life events: creation, birth, winning, nothingness, losing, separation, death. Their "I-Thou" empathetic relations with persons during these actual lived experiences and their own experiential-educational histories make "the between" of the nursing situation unique. Through in-touchness with self, authentic awareness and reflection on such experiences the human nurse comes to know. Humanistic nursing practice theory asks that the nurse describe what she comes to know: (1) the nurse's unique perspective and responses, (2) the other's knowable responses, and (3) the reciprocal call and response, the between, as they occur in the nursing situation.

Why Does Humanistic Nursing Practice Theory Ask That Existential Nursing Experience Be Described Phenomenologically?

There are many reasons. Philosophically and fundamentally the reason relates to how humanistic nursing perceives the purpose and aim of nursing. It views nursing as the ability to struggle with other man through peak experiences related to health and suffering in which the participants in the nursing situation are and become in accordance with their human potential. So, like Elie Wiesel, the novelist, who states in *One Generation After* that he writes to attest to events of human existence and to come to understand, humanistic nursing proposes that human forms of existence in nursing situations need attestation and that through describing, nurses will understand better and relate to man as man is. Thus the profession of nursing's service contribution to the community of man will ever become more.

The reasons for phenomenologically describing nursing are complex, interinfluential, and their ramifications are far reaching. Sequentially, the study and description of human phenomena presented in nursing situations will affect (1) the quality of the nursing situation, (2) man's general knowledge of the variation in human capacity for beingness, and (3) the development and form of the evolvement of nursing theory and science.

How Can Nurses Begin to Describe Humanistic Nursing Phenomenologically?

The process of how to describe nursing events entails deliberate responsible, conscious, aware, nonjudgmental existence of the nurse in the nursing situation followed by disciplined authentic reflection and description.

There are obvious common lived human experiences which if considered and wondered about, can advance a nurse's ability for phenomenological description. These experiences are easily cited, yet not easily plumbed. Often experiences such as anger, frustration, waiting, apathy, confusion, perplexity, questioning, surprise, conflict, headache, crying, laughing, joy are quickly theoretically and analytically interpreted, labeled, and dismissed. Examining, reexamining, mulling over, brooding on, and fussing with the situational context of these experiences as nonlabeled, raw human lived data can yield knowledge. Knowledge of the nurse's and her other's unique human existence in their on-going struggle becomes explicit. Superficial treatment of such human clues results in nonfulfillment of the realistic human possibilities of artful-scientific professional knowing and nursing.

Words are the major tools of phenomenological description. They are limited by our human ability to express, and yet they are the best tools we have for expressing the human condition. The novelist James Agee, in *Let Us Now Praise Famous Men*, says that though man or human relatedness never could be described perfectly it would be the greater crime not to try. This, too, is a basic premise of the humanistic nursing practice theory.

The words we use to describe and discuss this theory are easy words, everyday English words. We all know them. We, at times, narrow a word's meaning or make it more specific. Some problem is presented by words we are accustomed to using and hearing. Habit and our human fallibility can promote only superficial comprehension. Thoughtful awareness of the meaning of these same sequentially expressed words can convey the complexity of the never completely fathomable "all-at-onceness" of lived existence. This theory is expressed in terms like "existence confirming," "striving," "becoming," "relation," and "reflection." We intend such words to express the grasp with acceptance and recognition of human limitations while awesomely pondering the open-ended scope of each man's potential.

In time, with disciplined authentic reflective description, themes common and significant to nursing situations become apparent. They are then available for compilation, complementary synthesis, and on-going refinement. A nursing resource bank accrues: Not a bank that offers a map of how and what to do but rather one that further stimulates nurses' exploration and understanding.

THE EVOLVEMENT OF HUMANISTIC NURSING PRACTICE THEORY

Since 1960 Loretta T. Zderad and myself in dialogue, together, and with groups of nurses in graduate schools and in nursing service situations have reflected on, explored, and questioned our own and others' nursing situational experiences. Over this period we have come to value and appreciate the meaningfulness of these situations to man's existence. This constantly augmented our feelings of responsibility for contributing to these situations beneficially. Therefore, we looked at them for their tractability to research methodology. Their loadedness with variations, changes, uncontrollables, and our negative feelings about the implications of viewing human beings as predictable left the strict scientism of positivistic method wanting at this stage of man's knowing. We saw objectivity in nursing situations or our questions, nursing questions, in the realm of needing to now how man experienced his existence. This objectivity, or man's real lived reality paradoxically is subjectively ridden, man–world.

The existential literature dealt with substantive themes encountered in nursing experiences. As I previously stated this literature evolves from a phenomenological approach to studying being and existence. This approach to studying, describing, and developing an artistic science of nursing became Dr. Zderad's and my long-sought haven. All along existentialism and phenomenology had been ours 'and many nurses' "what" and "how." Now we had labels that were acceptable and reputable to many—most of all to ourselves.

2
FOUNDATIONS OF HUMANISTIC NURSING

Nursing is a response to the human situation. It comes into being under certain conditions—one human being needs a kind of help and another gives it. The meaning of nursing as a living human act is in the act itself. To understand it, therefore, it is necessary to consider nursing as an existent, a phenomenon occurring in the real world.

THE PHENOMENON OF NURSING

The phenomenon of nursing appers in many forms in the real lived world. It varies with the age of the patient, the pathology or disability, the kind and degree of help needed, the duration of the need for help, the patient's location and his potential for obtaining and using help, and the nurse's perception of the need and her capacities for responding to it. Nursing varies also in relation to the sociocultural context in which it occurs. Being one element in an evolving complex system of health care, nursing is continuously appearing in new specialized forms. As professionals, we are accustomed to viewing nursing as we practice it within these specialty contexts—for example, pediatric, medical, rehabilitation, intensive care, long-term care, community. There seems to be no end to the proliferation of diversifications. Even the attempts of practitioners to combine specialties give rise to new specialties, such as, community mental health nursing and child psychiatric nursing.

So it is difficult to focus on the phenomenon of nursing as an entity without having one's view colored by a particular clinical, functional, or societal context. Yet, if we can "bracket" (hold in abeyance) these adjectival labels and the preconceived viewpoints they signify, we can consider the thing itself, the act of nursing in its most simple and general appearance.

Well–Being and More–Being

In this most basic sense, then, disregarding the particular specialized forms in which it appears, the nursing act always is related to the health-illness quality of the human condition, or fundamentally, to a man's personal survival. This is not to say that all instances of nursing are matters of life and death, but rather that every nursing act has to do with the quality of a person's living and dying.

That nursing is related to health and illness is self-evident. How it is related is not so apparent. "Health" is valued as necessary for survival and is often proposed as the goal of nursing. There are, in actuality, many instances of nursing that could be described as "health restoring," "health sustaining," or "health promoting." Nurses engage in "health teaching" and "health supervision." On the other hand, there are instances in which health, taken in its narrowest meaning as freedom from disease, is not seen as an attainable goal, as evidenced, for example, in labels given to patients such as "terminal," "hopeless," and "chronic." Yet in actual practice these humans' conditions call forth some of the most complete, expert, total, beautiful nursing care. Nursing, then, as a human response, implies the valuing of some human potential beyond the narrow concept of health taken as absence of disease. Nursing's concern is not merely with a person's well-being but with his more-being, with helping him become more as humanly possible in his particular life situation.

Human Potential

Since nursing involves one human being helping another, the notion of humaneness has been associated traditionally with nursing. Nursing practice is criticized justifiably when it is not humane and is taken for granted or praised when it is. The expectation of humaneness is so ingrained in the concept of nursing that some nurses are surprised when it is acknowledged by patients. If a patient thanks them for their kindness, patience, or concern, these nurses reply, in their embarrassment, "Oh, that's part of my job."

However, to equate nursing's humanistic character solely with an overflowing of the milk of human kindness is a serious error of oversimplification. Such a limited view, in fact, is a dehumanizing denial of man's potentials. As a human transaction, the phenomenon of nursing contains all the human potentials and limtations of each unique participant. For instance, frustration, discouragement, anger, rejection, withdrawal, loneliness, aggression, impatience, envy, grief, despair, pain, and suffering are constituents of nursing, as well as tenderness, caring, courage, trust, joy, hope. In other words, since nursing is lived by humans, the "stuff" of nursing includes all possible responses of man—man needing and man helping—in his situation.

Intersubjective Transaction

Looking again at the phenomenon of nursing as it occurs in the real lived world, obviously it is always an interhuman event. Whenever nursing takes place two (or more) human beings are related in a shared situation. Each participates according to his own mode of being in the situation, that is, as a person nursing or as a person begin nursed. Since one is nursing and the other is being nursed, it follows that the essential character of the situation is "nurturance." In other words, the phenomenon of nursing involves nurturing, being nurtured, and a relation—the "between" in which or through which the nurturance occurs.

On reflection, it is obvious that nursing is an intersubjective transaction. Both persons, nurse and patient (client, family, group), necessarily participate in the proceedings. In this sense, they are *inter*dependent. Yet, they are both subjects, that is, each is the originator of human acts and of human responses to the other. In this sense, they are *in*dependent. The intersubjective transactional character of nursing cannot be escaped when one is experiencing the phenomenon, either as nurse or as patient. Consider for example, some of the most common nursing activities, such as, feeding and being fed, comforting and being comforted, giving and taking medications. Although this intersubjectivity is unmistakably known in experience, it is extremely difficult to conceptualize and convey it to others. It rarely is found in descriptions of nursing, and to the unfortunate extent that it is missing, the descriptions are not true to life.

In real life, nursing phenomena may be experienced from the reference points of nurturing, of being nurtured, or of the nurturing process in the "between." For instance, the nurse may describe comfort as an experience of comforting another person; the patient, as an experience of being comforted. However, while each has experienced something within himself, he also has experienced something of the "between," namely, the message or meaning of the "comforting–being comforted" process. This essential interhuman dimension of nursing is beyond and yet within the technical, procedural, or interactional elements of the event. It is a quality of being that is expressed in the doing.

Being and Doing

As an intersubjective, transactional experience, nursing necessarily involves both a mode of being and a doing of something. The being and doing are interrelated so inextricably that it is difficult, even distorting, to speak of one without the other. Descriptions of nursing, however, often focus primarily (sometimes exclusively) on the doing aspect of the process, on the nursing techniques or procedures. The observable acts are more easily discerned and discussed. They can be measured, counted, and charted. Yet, in the actual interhuman experience of nursing the weight of being is felt. Presence and the effect of one's presence can be known much more vividly than they can be described. Still, not to attempt to describe them is to present only a half, or perhaps less than half, of the nursing picture.

When a nurse refers to a nurse–patient interaction during which a change in the patient's condition or behavior was noted, one hoping to get a description of nursing may ask, "What did you do?" Often the answer is a description of a manual action or a verbal interchange. Sometimes the nurse responds, "Nothing, I was just there." Perhaps it is the question that is wrong. The respondent usually interprets "doing" in a limited sense. In reality, everything the nurse does is colored by the character of her being in the situation. The nursing act itself is a behavioral expression of the nurse's state of being, for example, concerned, fatigued, hurried, confident, hopeless.

Furthermore, there is a kind of being, a "being with" or a "being there," that is really a kind of doing for it involves the nurse's active presence. To "be with" in this fuller sense requires turning one's attention toward the patient, being aware of and open to the here and now shared siuation, and communicating one's availability.

Whether the nursing act is verbal, or manual, or both, a silent glance, or physical presence, some degree of intersubjectivity is involved and warrants recognition. To become more aware of and explore more fully this essential constituent of nursing we need to focus on the participants' modes of being in the situation. Rather than ask the nurse, "What did you do in the nurse–patient situation?" we ought to ask, "What happened between you?"

HUMANISTIC NURSING

When the meaning of nursing is sought by scrutinizing the phenomenon, that is, by examining the nursing event itself as it occurs in real life, one finds nursing embedded within the human context. As a nurturing response of one person to another in need, it aims at the development of human potential, at well-being and more-being. As something that happens between people, it reflects all the human potential and limitations of the persons involved. As an intersubjective transaction, it holds the possibility for both persons to effect and be affected, the possibility for both to become more. At its very base, then, nursing is humanistic. It is, at once, man's expression of and his striving for survival and further development in community.

In a way, to specify nursing as humanistic seems redundant. In view of its source and goals how could it be otherwise? However, the term "humanistic nursing" was coined thoughtfully and used purposely here to designate a particular nursing approach. Not only does the term signify full recognition of nursing's human foundation and meaning but it also points the direction for nursing's necessary development. What is proposed here is the enrichment of nursing by exploring and expanding its relations to its human context.

Authentic Commitment

When it is genuinely humanistic, nursing is an expression, a living out, of the nurse's authentic commitment. It is an existential engagement directed toward nurturing human potential. The humanistic nurse values nursing as a situation in which the necessary conditions for such human actualization exist and is open to the possibilities in the intimately shared nurse–patient here and now.

Humanistic nursing calls for an existential involvement, that is, an active presence with the whole of the nurse's being. This involved presence is personal and professional. It is personal—a live act stemming from this unique, individual nurse. It is a chosen human response freely given; it cannot be assigned or programmed. The involvement is professional—goal directed. It is based on an art-science; it is held accountable.

Anyone familiar with typical hectic nursing situations could justifiably question the actual attainability of such an existential involvement. It goes wothout saying that it would be humanly impossible for a nurse to be wholly present to numerous patients for eight hours a day. But any nurse who has experienced moments of genuine presence in the nurse–patient situation will attest to their reality and to the fact that it is these beautiful moments that give meaning to nursing. In terms of actual practice, then, it is more realistic to think of humanistic nursing as occurring in various degrees. It may be more useful, in fact, to consider humanistic nursing a goal worth striving for; or an attitude that strengthens one's perseverance toward attaining the difficult goal; or fundamentally, a major value shaping one's nursing practice.

Process—Choice and Intersubjectivity

For the process of nursing to be truly humanistic it must bear out, that is, be a lived expression of, the nurse's recognition and valuing of nursing as an opportunity for the development of the human person. To this end, humanistic nursing process echos existential themes related to a person's becoming through choice and intersubjectivity.

Existentially speaking, man is his choices. This does not mean that a man can be anything he chooses. Naturally, each individual is unique, having his own particular potentials and limitations. Nor is this view a denial of the forces of unconscious motivation and habit. It does not imply that all of a person's actions result from totally conscious deliberations. By saying, ''I am my choices,'' I mean I am this here and now person because in my past life I took particular paths in preference to others; of the possibilities open to me, I actualized certain ones.

In this sense, I am my history, I am what I am, what I have become. But I am also what I am not, what I have not become. I am a nurse, this unique here and now nurse with particular experience, knowledge, skills, and values; without other experience, knowledge, skills, and values. Through self-reflection I know that I have changed, I have experienced growth from within. I know myself as a being capable of becoming more, capable of actualizing my possibilities, my self. So I am my choices not only in terms of my past but also in regard to my future, my possibilities.

Man is an individual being necessarily related to other men in time and space. As every man is beholden to other men for his birth and development, interdependence is inherent in the human situation. In this sense, human existence is coexistence. The deeper significance of this truth has been recognized and elucidated by many thinkers, especially those in the existential stream. Over and over, their writings reveal the paradoxical tension of being human: each man is, at once, independent, a unique individual and interdependent, a necessarily related being. As Wilfrid Desan says, referring to man as subsistent relation, "He is towards-the-other but he is not-the-other."[1]

Furthermore, as Martin Buber and Gabriel Marcel maintain, it is actually through his relations with other men that a man becomes, that his unique individuality is actualized. To know myself as "individual" is to experience myself as this particular unique here-and-now person and other than that there-and-now person. Or in other words, to know myself as me is to see myself in relation to and distant from other selves. As Buber so beautifully states, "It is from one man to another that the heavenly bread of self-being is passed."[2]

Logically, it follows that the possibility for self-confirmation exists in any intersubjective situation. However, in everyday life this self-confirmation is experienced to different degrees or on different levels in interhuman relating. Since both persons are independent subjects acting with their human capacity for disclosing or enclosing themselves, there is no guarantee that the availability and presence necessary for a genuine confirming encounter will come forth. Presence, the gift of one's self, cannot be seized or called forth by demand, it can only be given freely and be invoked or evoked.

Since man becomes more through his choices and the aim of nursing is to help man toward well-being or more-being, the humanistic nursing effort is directed toward increasing the possibilities of making responsible choices. Such choice involves, in the first place, an openness to and an awareness of one's own situation. A choice is a response to possibility. Therefore, one must first recognize that possibilities or alternatives exist. This openness to options is experienced as a freedom to choose as well as a freedom from the bonds of habit and stereotyped response, from routine, from the veils of the obvious. It means getting in touch with one's experience, one's subjective–objective world. As one becomes more acutely aware of his personal freedom of choice, there arises concurrently an awareness of the quality of choice, of the responsibility that is always implied in the freedom. Then follows reflective consideration of one's unique situation with its possible alternatives and an examination of the values inherent in them. Finally, the act of choosing is expressed in a response to the situation with a willingness to accept the responsibility for its foreseeable consequences. Through this experience the person becomes aware of himself as an individual. As a subject choosing freely and responsibly, he knows himself as distinct from and yet related to others.

Nursing, being an intersubjective transaction, presents an occasion for both persons, patient and nurse, to experience the process of making responsible choices. Through living this process in nursing situations, the nurse develops her own potential for responsible choosing. The satisfaction, often in the form

[1] Wilfred Desan, *The Planetary Man,* Vol. I, *A Noetic Prelude to a United World* (New York: The Macmillan Company, 1972). p. 37.

[2] Martin Buber, "Distance and Relation," trans. Ronald Gregor Smith, in *The Knowledge of Man,* ed. Maurice Friedman (New York: Harper & Row, Publishers, 1965), p. 71.

of a sense of vitality and strength, that is felt in making responsible competent professional judgments reinforces the habit. In personally coming to experientially appreciate the growth promoting character of responsible choosing, the nurse may more readily recognize the value of such experiences for any person, including the one currently labeled "patient." The humanistic nurse, therefore, is alert to opportunities for the patient to exercise his freedom of choice within the limits of safe and sound practice. She is constantly assessing his capabilities and needs and encourages his maximum participation in his own health care program. Through coexperiencing and supporting the process in the patient's experience from his point of view, the nurse nurtures his human potential for responsible choosing. Both patient and nurse become more through making responsible choices in the intersubjective, transactional nursing situation.

Theory and Practice

The term "humanistic nursing" refers to a kind of nursing practice and its theoretical foundations. The two are so interrelated that it is difficult, in fact even somewhat distorting, to speak exclusively of either the practice or the theory of humanistic nursing. When, for the sake of clarity or emphasis, discussion is focused on either the practical or the theoretical realm, thoughts of the other realm cast their shadows on the fringes. For in our view, for the process of nursing to be truly humanistic means that the nurse is involved as an experiencing, valuing, reflecting, conceptualizing human person. From the other side, the theory of humanistic nursing is derived from actual practice, that is, from being with and doing with the patient. "Theory," says R. D. Laing, "is the articulated vision of experience."[3]

Humanistic nursing is not a matter solely of doing but also of being. The humanistic nurse is open to the reality of the situation in the existential sense. She is available with her total being in the nurse–patient situation. This involves a living out of the nurturing, intersubjective transaction with all of one's human capacities which include a response to the experienced reality. Man is able to set his world at a distance as an independent opposite and enter into relation with it. In fact, according to Buber, this is what distinguishes existence as human. It is man's special way of being.[4] For nursing to be humanistic in this full sense of the term requires being and doing in the situation and subsequently setting the experienced reality at a distance (that is, objectifying it) and entering into relation with it. The nurse's reflective response to her lived world may take the shape of any form of human dialogue with reality, such as, science, art, or philosophy.

Viewed existentially, every nursing event is unique, a live intersubjective transaction colored and formed by the individual participants. Although the event is ephemeral, the resultant experiential knowledge is lasting and cumulative. So

[3] R.D. Laing, *The Politics of Experience* (New York: Ballantine Books, 1967), p. 23.
[4] Buber, *The Knowledge of Man,* p. 60.

from the nurse's daily commonplace grows a body of clinical wiscom. The need for describing nursing phenomena, for expressing and conceptualizing lived nursing worlds, is basic to the theoretical and actual development of humanistic nursing. In summary, we contend that humanistic nursing practice necessarily involves the conceptualization of that practice and an examination of its inherent values and that humanistic nursing theory must be derived from nurses' lived experience. The interwoven theory and practice are reciprocally enlightening.

Framework—The Human Situation

It is easy to recognize the intrinsic interrelatedness of humanistic nursing theory and practice and the consequent necessity for their concurrent development. It is even quite easy to take the next steps of valuing such development and committing oneself to the task. But then the question arises: Where to begin?

Humanistic nursing is concerned with what is basically nursing, that is, with the phenomenon of nursing wherever it occurs regardless of its specialized clinical, functional, or sociocultural form. So its domain includes any or all nursing situations. And within this domain, since humanistic nursing is an intersubjective transaction aimed at nurturing well-being and more-being, its "stuff" includes all possible human and interhuman responses. To conceive of so limitless a universe for study is at once exhilarating and overwhelming. How can one get a handle on the nursing universe? Is it possible to envision an inclusive frame that would allow an orderly, systematic, and hopefully productive approach to the development of humanistic nursing?

The key is to return again to the source, to look at the phenomenon of nursing as it occurs in real life. From this perspective, the human situation sets the stage where nursing is lived. The major dimensions of humanistic nursing, then, may be derived from this situation. Existentially, man is an incarnate being always becoming in relation with men and things in a world of time and space. The nursing situation is a particular kind of human situation in which the interhuman relating is purposely directed toward nurturing the well-being or more-being of a person with perceived needs related to the health–illness quality of living. The elements of the frame, based on this view of humanistic nursing, would include incarnate men (patient and nurse) meeting (being and becoming) in a goal directed (nurturing well-being and more-being) intersubjective transaction (being with and doing with) occurring in time and space (measured and as lived by patient and nurse) in a world of men and things. In other words, the inexhaustible richness of lived nursing wourlds could be explored freely, imaginatively, and creatively in any direction suggested by the dimensions of this open framework. It allows for a variety of angular views.

For example, in terms of man as incarnate, it is certainly not new for nurses to focus on man's bodily existence. Naturally, one of nursing's basic concerns always has been care of people's physical needs. To view nursing from the perspective of the human situation, however, is to see beyond physical care, beyond the categorization of man as a biopsychosocial organism. The focus is on the person's unique being and becoming in his situation.

Every man is inserted into the common world of men and things through his own unique body. Through it he affects the world and the world affects him. Through it he develops his own unique personal private world. When a person's bodily functions change during illness *the* world and *his* world change for him. The nurse needs to consider how the patient experiences his lived world. Ordinary things which nurses simply take for granted, such as, hospital noises or odors, touching, bathing, feeding, sleep or meal schedules, may have very different meaning for individual patients. They may or may not be experienced as nurturing in a particular person's lived world.

In the humanistic perspective the nurse also is viewed as a human person, as a being in a body rather than merely as a function or a doer of activities. Conscious recognition of this fact opens many areas for exploration. Obviously, the nurse's actions (her being with and doing with), that affect the patient's world, are expressed through her body. How is nurturance communicated and actually effected through nursing activities? From the other side, consider the nurse as being affected by the world through her body. What depths of "nursing content" could we fathom if we accepted the existential dictum that "the body knows?" Would we dismiss so lightly those gems of clinical wisdom nurses attribute disparagingly to "gut reaction," "unscientific intuition," or "years of experience"? Would we value serious exploration and extraction of these natural resources in the nursing world?

The framework suggests, further, the possibilities of exploring the development of human potential, both patient's and nurse's, as it occurs in the unique domain of nursing's intersubjective transactions. What human resources are called forth in the shared situations during which nurses coexperience and cosearch with patients the varied meanings of being and becoming over the entire range of life from birth to death? How does it occur? What is the process? What promotes well-being or becoming more when facing life, suffering, death? For the patient? For the nurse? What knowledge gained through the study of nursing, a particular form of the human situation, could be contributed to the general body of human sciences?

Finally, within this framework, all the phenomena experienced in the nursing situation could be explored in relation to their attributes of time and space. More specifically, from an existential perspective, the focus would be directed toward the significance of lived time and space, that is, time and space as experienced by the patient and/or the nurse, and as shared intersubjectively. For example, waiting, silence, chronicity, emergency, positioning a patient in bed, moving through space in a wheelchair, crutchwalking, pacing, could be considered from the standpoint of the patient's experienced space and time, or from the nurse's, or as a shared event. Explorations of this kind could provide valuable insights into important nursing phenomena, such as, presence, empathy, comfort, timing.

The human situation, then, is the ground within which nursing takes form. As such, it provides a framework for approaching the study and development of humanistic nursing. As an angular view, it holds the focus on the basic question underlying nursing practice: Is this particular intersubjective, transactional nursing event humanizing or dehumanizing?

CONCLUSION

This chapter explored the foundations of humanistic nursing. The discussion flowed naturally, perhaps unavoidably, into the realm of meta-nursing. "Naturally," for the humanistic nursing appraoch is itself an outgrowth of the critical examination of nursing as an experienced phenomenon. From this existential perspective of nursing as a living human act, the meaning of nursing is found in the act itself, in nursing's relation to its human context.

Reflection on nursing as it is lived in the real world revealed its existential, nurturing, intersubjective, transactional character. The process of humanistic nursing stemming from the nurse's authentic commitment is a kind of being with and doing with. It aims at the development of human potential through intersubjectivity and responsible choosing.

The actualization of humanistic nursing is dependent on the concurrent development of its practice and theoretical foundations by practicing nurses. An open framework derived from the human situation was offered to suggest possible dimensions of humanistic nursing practice that could be described and articulated into a body of theory.

Nurses who have considered this humanistic nursing approach in terms of their daily practice have felt at home in the ideas. The conceptualizations fit their personal nursing experience. If there is any strangeness in the approach, it is perhaps that it does not follow the contours of the clinical specialties to which we have grown so accustomed that they may be more ruts than roads. This is not to say that humanistic nursing is opposed to clinical specialization in nursing. In fact, clinical nursing, as it exists in any form, is its very heart and base. Humanistic nursing is not compartmentalized into clinical (or functional, or sociocultural) specialties because it applies in all clinical areas. It is, in the most basic sense, cross-clinical. This may be the great advantage of humanistic nursing. By orienting its explorations ontologically, it may foster genuine cross-clincal studies of nursing phenomena. If nurses with highly developed abilities in particular forms of nursing would struggle together in collaborative cross-clinical studies of nursing phenomena, specialization would serve to advance rather than fragment all nursing.

3

HUMANISTIC NURSING: A LIVED DIALOGUE

The meaning of humanistic nursing is found in the human act itself, that is, in the phenomenon of nursing as it is experienced in the everyday world. Therefore, the interrelated practical and theoretical development of humanistic nursing is dependent on nurses experiencing, conceptualizing, and sharing their unique angular views of their unique lived nursing worlds. An open framework suggesting dimensions for such exploration was derived from a consideration of the phenomenon of nursing within its basic context, namely, the human situation. The elements of this humanistic nursing framework include incarnate men (patient and nurse) meeting (being and becoming) in a goal-directed (nurturing well-being and more-being), intersubjective transaction (being with and doing with) occurring in time and space (as measured and as lived by patient and nurse) in a world of men and things.

The framework offers a little security by providing some reference points for the exploration. However, what is gained in clairty by conceptual abstraction is lost from the flavor of the actual experience. Like a weather map that statically represents major factors and currents in their interrelatedness, the framework discloses a nexus of elements. But it is as far from the real phenomenon of nursing with its pains and suffering and comforting and joys and hopes as the weather map is from real weather with its wind and rain and heat and cold. This chapter is concerned with the same basic framework of humanistic nursing but seen in an enlivened form. To inspirit its constructs the search must return again to the existential source, to the nursing situation as it is lived.

When I reflect on an act of mine (no matter how simple or complex) that I can unhesitatingly label ''nursing,'' I become aware of it as goal-directed (nurturing) being with and doing with another. The intersubjective or interhuman element, ''the between,'' runs through nusing interactions like an underground stream conveyting the nutrients of healing and growth. In everyday practice, we are usually so involved with the immediate demands of our ''being with and

21

doing with" the patient that we do not focus on the overshadowed plane of "the between." However, occasionally, in beautiful moments, the interhuman currents are so strong that they flood our conscious awareness. Such rare and rewarding moments of mutual presence remind us of the elusive ever-present "between."

From these epiphanic episodes in our personal nursing experience, we have certain and immediate knowledge of intersubjectivity. Through our experience, too, we know that both humanizing and dehumanizing effects can result from human interactions. Therefore, it is essential for the development of humanistic nursing to explore and describe its intersubjective character.

Although many nurses have agreed in principle about the importance of this work, they also have expressed the feelings of frustration and discouragement attending it. There are real difficulties involved in attempting to describe something so real yet so nebulous as "the between." The descriptions must be derived from our own real nursing experiences. This means that we must develop habits of conscious awareness of experience, of recall, and of reflection. Then we must struggle with our language finding the words in our physically and technologically oriented vocabularies, perhaps even creating terms, to convey the substance and flavor of the experience of intersubjectivity.

Furthermore, description of the intersubjective quality of nursing is difficult because of its peculiar pervasiveness. Whether it is consciously recognized or not, it is part of every nursing transaction. However, to consider and explore intersubjectivity solely as a component or consitituent of nursing, even a necessarily inherent or an essential one, would be to see it out of true perspective. The "between" is more than a factor or facet of nursing; it is the basic relation in which and through which nursing can occur. So the question remains. How can our experiences, our angular views, our glimpses of this foundation, this necessary means of nursing, be conceptualized and shared?

Once while relfecting on the nature of nursing against a background of notions about intersubjectivity drawn from experience and literature and testing them against my own real life experiences of nursing, I suddenly saw that *nursing itself is a particular form of human dialogue.* This insight occurred to me with clarity, conviction, and all the force of a brand new idea. It was so obvious, so distinct, so simple, so clearly a central intuition that could illuminate the phenomenon of nursing from within. I experienced the idea as fresh and excitingly full of promise.

Yet, when I said it out loud, "Nursing is dialogue," the words seemed too meager to convey the true meaning of the idea and its real significance. There was, furthermore, an annoying shadow of familiarity lurking about it. It was almost as if I had expressed something similar previously. At first, I hesitated to share this insight with others for fear they would extinguish it by saying, "of course, everyone knows that," or "I've heard you say something like that before." Still, I experienced it as an idea I *had* to express. Moved by the pressure of feelings of responsibility and desire to share, in 1973 I wrote a paper, "The Dialogue Called Nursing."

In retrospect, that paper has the marks of a hesitant beginning, restrained by cautious statements and supposedly protective references to existential literature. Dissatisfaction with it prompted further rethinking and revision. Searching through my files during this process, I found, to my great surprise, some notes on the dialogic nature of nursing written by myself three and six years previously. In fact, a three-year-old note contained the very title, "Dialogue Called Nursing"! Now, how is it possible to grasp a truth and then "forget" that one knows it and later meet and grasp the old truth again as new? The difference in these experiences of knowing, for me at least in this case, is that now I know as if from the inside out that nursing is dialogical. The idea seems to have sprouted out of the lived phenomenon, to have broken forth from the ground of experience, as opposed to having been concluded in my earlier "intellectual," "theoretical," or "philosophical" ponderings. But how did the earlier idea, the conclusion that nursing is dialogical, become a live option for me? Why did it appeal to me? How did it come to make sense in the first place if not because of my experience?

The concept and the actual experience revitalize each other. Perhaps this is the value of an existentially grounded insight; it has a kind of durability resulting from its continuous rejuvenation by the interplay of experiencing and conceptualizing. Some old ideas are always new. In this spirit, this chapter looks again at humanistic nursing as lived dialogue.

LIVED DIALOGUE

The central insight (intuition or idea) from which this exploration grows is this: nursing itself is a form of human dialogue. I mean that the phenomenon of nursing, that is, the nurturing, intersubjective transaction, the event lived or experienced by the participants in the everyday world, is a dialogue.

Much has been written about dialogue and, as the word is now in vogue, it is being used in different ways. Here, the term "dialogue" is used to denote a broader concept than the typical dicionary definition of dialogue as "a conversation between two or more persons or between characters in a drama or novel." It is used in the existential sense. It implies an "ontological sphere," in Buber's terms, or the "realm of being" to which Marcel refers. Here it refers to a *lived* dialogue, that is, to a particular form of intersubjective relating. This may be understood in terms of seeing the other person as a distinct unique individual and entering into relation with him. In other words, nursing is a dialogical mode of being in an intersubjective situation.

As in common usage, here also, the term "dialogue" implies communication, but in a much more general sense. It is not restricted to the notion of sending and receiving messages verbally and nonverbally. Rather, dialogue is viewed as communication in terms of call and response.

Nursing implies a special kind of meeting of human persons. It occurs in response to a perceived need related to the health-illness quality of the human condition. Within that domain, which is shared by other health professions, nursing is directed toward the goal of nurturing well-being and more-being (human potential). Nursing, therefore, does not involve a merely fortuitous encounter but rather one in which there is purposeful call and response. In this vein, humanistic nursing may be considered as a special kind of lived dialogue.

NURSING VIEWED AS DIALOGUE

These considerations of the dialogical character of nursing will be more fruitful if they are related to some concrete nursing experience. Reflect for a moment on your daily nursing practice. Recall an encounter, a specific interaction with a patient (client). Try to remember the details. Where were you? What time of day was it? Who was present? What was your state of being—what were you feeling, thinking, doing? How did the interaction begin? What happened between you? What was felt, said, done? What was left unsaid, undone? How did the interaction end or close? How long did the flavor last? Now keep this concrete instance of your lived nursing reality in mind and let it raise its questions in the following exploration.

Meeting

The act of nursing involves a meeting of human persons. As was noted above, it is a special or particular kind of meeting because it is purposeful. Both patient and nurse have a goal or expectation in mind. The intersubjective transaction, therefore, has meaning for them; the event is experienced in light of their goal(s). Or in other words, the living human act of nursing is formed by its purpose. Its goal-directedness colors the attributes and process of the nursing dialogue.

When a nurse and patient come together in a nursing situation, their meeting may be expected or planned by one or both or it may be unexpected by one or both. In any case, the goal or purpose of nursing holds. Even in a spontaneous interaction where they have met only by chance, in a health care facility or any place where one is identified as patient and the other as nurse, there is an implicit expectation that the nurse will extend herself in a helpful way if the patient needs assistance. If the meeting is planned or expected, this factor influences the dialogue. Each comes with feelings aroused by anticipation of the event, for example anxiety, fear, dread, hope, pleasure, waiting, impatience, dependence, hostility, responsibility.

Another factor experienced in their meeting is the amount of choice or control either nurse or patient had over their coming together. In today's complex health care systems, a nurse may be assigned to care for a particular patient, or for persons in an area or unit, or may be called into service through a registry, or may be approached directly by a patient. From the other side, the patient also experiences varying degrees of control over his meetings with nurses depending on the system in which the health care is offered, his location, his financial means, and so forth. So when a patient and nurse do meet in a given instance, each comes to the situation bearing remnants of feeling of having caused or not having caused this encounter with this particular individual. (Of course, even in the most de-individualized systems the nurse and/or patient can still control their meetings to some extent, for example, avoidance by the nurse being too busy or avoidance by the patient feigning sleep.)

The patient and the nurse are two unique individuals meeting for a purpose. In the existential sense, each of these persons is his choice, each is his history. Each comes to meet the other with all that he is and all that he is not at this moment in this place. Each comes as a particular incarnate being. Each is a specific being in a specific body through which he affects the other and the world and through which he is affected by them. This nurse who uses her eyes, ears, nose, hands, her body, this way here and now meets this patient whose body in this condition serves him this way here and now.

Furthermore, both the patient and the nurse have the human capacity for disclosing or enclosing themselves. So they have some control over the quality of their meeting by choosing how and how much to be open with and to be open to the other. Their openness is influenced by their views of the purpose of the meeting. In general, the patient expects to receive help and the nurse expects ot give it. However, their views may differ on the precise need and the kind of help to be given.

Also, although the nurse and the patient have the same goal, that is, well-being and more-being, they have different modes of being in the shared situation. One's purpose is to nurture; the other's is to be nurtured. This difference in the perspectives from which they approach the meeting is reflectd in the kind and degree of their openness to each other.

In describing their experiences nurses often have revealed that they are open to patients in a certain way. This is evident when nurse and patient meet. The nurse may have prior knowledge of the patient, perhaps even an image of him drawn from case history, charts, tour of duty reports, and so forth; or she may meet him as a total stranger. But when they come together, the nurse sees "the patient as a whole." This global apprehension is not experienced as an additive summation but rather as a gestalt. It may result in a very clear "picture" of the patient's condition with nursing action initiated almost before the picture registers in full conscious awareness. Or the perception may be imprecise yet strong that "something is wrong." From these experiences one may infer that a nurse's openness involves being open to what is and to what is not in the patient's state of being as weighed against some notion (or standard) of what "ought" to be, with the intention of doing something about the difference. Thus, the nurse is open-as-a-helper to the patient. This kind of openness is a quality that characterizes the humanistic nursing dialogue. Of course, every nurse-patient meeting differs, for each participant comes to the situation as the unique individual he is, with his own expectations and capacities for giving and taking help.

When these factors are considered in terms of an actual personal nursing experience (for instance, the example recalled above by the reader), they highlight a tension in the lived nursing world. The meeting through which the nursing dialogue is initiated and consequently is possible is, to a certain extent, out of the nurse's control. She is assigned to approach or she approaches the patient in terms of her function. In this sense, "the nurse" is synonymous with the function "nursing." Yet she experiences each meeting as herself—a unique individual person, this here-and-now being in this body responding in this situation. She is at once a replaceable cog in a wheel of an incomprehensibly complex system and a unique human being sharing most intimately in another's search for the meanings of suffering, living, dying. Can these two world views be reconciled? How can they be lived in the nursing dialogue?

Relating

As a human response to a person in need, the nursing act is necessarily an intersubjective transaction. Or to put it in other words, regardless of the complexity of need and/or response, when nurse and patient meet in the event of nursing both have "to do" with each other. Since both are human, their doing with means being with. (Reflect for a moment on the personally experienced patient encounter you recalled at the beginning of this exploration. Relive it and see clearly again that the nursing dialogue involves being with and doing with the patient.)

Men can do with and be with each other because they are able to see others and things as distinct from themselves and enter into relation with them. What distinguishes the human situation is that men can enter into a dialogue with reality. They have a capacity for for internal relationships, for knowing themselves and their worlds within themselves, they can relate as subject to object (for example, as knower to thing known) and as subject to subject, that is, as person to person. Both types of relationships are essential for genuine human existence.

It is natural, in fact unavoidable, for man to relate to his world as subject to object. How could a person survive even one day without knowing and using objects? Therefore, man's abilities to abstract, objectify, conceptualize, categorize, and so forth, are necessary tor everyday living. Even beyond this, the human capacity for relating to the other as object is basic to the advancement of mankind for it underlies science, art, and philosophy. It is simply one way of being human.

Another mode of relating is open to men. Whenever two persons are present to each other as human beings, the possibility of intersubjective dialogue exists. Since both are subjects with the capabilities for internal relationships, they can be open, available, and knowable to each other. They can know each other within themselves. Furthermore, they can be truly with each other in the intersubjective realm because while maintaining their own unique identities, they can participate in an interior union. Intersubjective relating is also necessary for human existence. For it is through his relationships with other men that a person develops his human potential and becomes a unique individual.

Nursing, being an interhuman event, has within it possibilities for various types and degrees of relationships. Both nurse and patient can view themselves and the other as objects and as subjects or in any variation or combination of these ways. A person can view and relate to another person as an object, for instance as a mere function ("patient," "nurse," "supervisor," "medicine nurse," "admitting nurse," "administration") or as a case or type ("schizophrenic," "cardiac," "outpatient," "readmission," "bed patient," "wheelchair patient," "total care patient," "terminal patient"). Such subject-object or "I-It" relationships differ essentially from subject-subject or "I-Thou" relationships.

As the derivation of the term indicates, an object is something placed before or opposite; it is anything that can be apprehended intellectually. Through objectivication the object is de-individualized and therefore made replaceable for the purpose of study by any other object with the same properties. It is indifferent to the act by which it is thought and, therefore, the subject studying the object may also be replaced by a similar subject.

Although it is possible to view a person as an object, persons and things are necessarily different kinds of objects. A thing, as object, is open to a subject's scrutiny, while a person, as object, can make himself knowable or set up barriers to objectification. He can keep his thoughts to himself, remain silent, or deliberately conceal some of his qualities.

Through the scientific objective approach, that is, subject-object relating, it is possible to gain certain knowledge about a person; through intersubjective, that is, subject-subject relating, it is possible to know a person in his unique individuality. Thus, both subject-subject and subject-object relationships are essential to the clinical nursing process. Both are integral elements of humanistic nursing.

Presence

In the nursing world, as in the world at large, human encounters may range from the trivial to the extremely significant. Within a day's work, the nurse may experience many levels of intersubjectivity from the lowest level of being called on as a function or being used as an object, to the other end of the scale of being recognized as a presence or a thou in genuine dialogue.

Nursing activities bring a nurse and patient into close physical proximity, but his in itself does not guarantee genuine intersubjectivity in which a man relates to another person as a "presence" rather than an object. A presence cannot be grasped or seized like an object. It cannot be demanded or commanded; it only can be welcomed or rejected. In a sense, it lies beyond comprehension and can only be invoked or evoked.

There is a quality of unpredictableness or spontaneity about genuine dialogue. A nurse may be going through her daily activities, functioning effectively, relating humanely, when suddenly she is stopped by something in the patient, perhaps a look of fear, a tug at her sleeve, a moan, a reaching for her hand, a question, emptiness. In a suspenseful pause two persons hover between their private worlds and the realm of intersubjectivity. Two humans stand on the brink of the between for a precious moment filled with promise and fear. With my hand on the doorknob to open myself from within, I hesitate—should I, will I let me out, let him in? Time is suspended, then moves again as I move with resolve to recognize, to give testimony to the other presence.

Thus, for genuine dialogue to occur there must be a certain openness, a receptivity, readiness, or availability. The open or available person reveals himself as "present." This is not the same as being attentive; a listener may be attentive and still refuse to give himself. Visible actions do not necessarily signify presence so it cannot be proven. But it can be revealed directly and unmistakably in a glance, a touch, a tone of voice. (I can only ask you to substantiate this statement with your own experience.) Availability implies, therefore, not only being at the other's disposal but also being with him with the whole of oneself. Furthermore, it involves a reciprocity. The other is also seen as a presence, as a person rather than an object, such as a function or a case.

As was discussed earlier, the nursing dialogue occurs within the domain of health and illness and has a purpose in the minds of the participants. Nursing is a lived dialogue (a being with and doing with) aimed at nurturing well-being and more-being. This fact of goal-directedness modifies or characterizes dialogical presence. As a nurse I try to be open to the other as a person, a presence, and to be available to the other. Yet, when I reflect upon my presence, I realize that my openness is an openness to a "person-with-needs" and my availability is an "availability-in-a-helping-way." By comparison, my experiences of openness and availbaility in social, family, or friend relationships and in nurse-patient relationships differ. In the later, I find myself responding with a kind of "professional reserve." While it is true that what I conceive of as "professional" and the degree of "reserve" has varied over the years and from patient to patient, nevertheless, it is always a factor influencing the tone of my lived dialogue of nursing.

It is the qualitative differences in the various experiences of presence that deserve, yet almost defy, description. For instance, the presence seems to have a different quality of *intimacy*. It is not experienced as less intense or less deep in the nurse-patient relationship, but as somehow colored by a sense of responsibility or regard for what is seen as the patient's vulnerability. At times I am aware of a shadow of "holding back" in terms of what I consider "nurturing" or "therapeutically appropriate" at a given moment. As a nurse, I find my presence flows through a filter of therapeutic tact.

Or again, the *mutuality* of presence may be experienced in the nurse-patient situation. At times I become consciously and acutely aware of the reciprocal flow of openness in the dialogue. It is as strong, definite, immediate, and total as in other dialogical relationships and yet it is somehow different. It is felt as a flow between two persons with different modes of begin in the shared situation. My reason for being there, to nurture, and his, to be nurtured, bob into my consciousness like buoys marking the channel of openness.

Often in nursing it is necessary to focus my attention on some aspect of the patient's body or behavior. The patient may or may not have the same focus of attention. At least momentarily then, or even for a prolonged period, I place some aspect of the patient before or opposite myself (that is, objectify it). And to the extent that this detail absorbs my attention, I lose my sight of and my relatedness to the whole person who happens to be the patient. While I know this focusing on details to be a necessary step in the nursing process, sometimes I find myself abruptly refocusing my attention on the whole person with almost a twinge of guilt for having abandoned him. (Patients have described this uncomfortable intersubjective experience as feeling "looked at" or "watched " by staff.) At other times, on reflection, I find my attention was oscillating between the detail and the person, or focusing on both relating one to the other. From these experiences it is evident that dialogical presence is complicated in the nursing situation. It is inhibited when the focus of attention (of one or both participants) is on the patient's body itself or on his behavior. Yet the body is an integral part of the person and his behavior is an expression of his mode of existence or his way of being in the world. Man is an embodied being, and the nurse, in nurturing the patient's well-being and more-being, must relate to him and his body in their mysterious interrelatedness.

Call and Response

The dialogical character of nursing may be explored further by considering it in the general sense of a call and response. Nursing is a purposefull call and response, that is, it is related to some particular kind of help in the domain of health and illness. A patient calls for a nurse with the expectation of being cared for, of having his need met. He is asking for something. A nurse responds to a patient for the purpose of meeting his need, of caring for him. The nurse expects to be needed.

In reflecting on nursing experiences, it becomes obvious that the call and response in the nursing dialogue goes both ways for nursing is transactional. Both patient and nurse call and respond. The pattern of the dialogue is complex. It continues over time, from moments to years, in an ongoing sequence that either patient or nurse may begin, interrupt, resume, or end. For instance, the patient turns on his call light to ask for something. This is not only a call but also a response to the nurse's previously stated suggestion that he use the signal if he needs her help. Or again, a nurse may stop and talk with a patient during a chance meeting recalling that he previously had expressed feelings of loneliness, boredom, pain, or joy. Also, other persons or events may interrupt or end a nursing dialogue. For instance, the nurse is called away to help in another situation, the patient is discharged on the nurse's day off, the patient expires.

Furthermore, the call and response are not only sequential but also simultaneous. In this live dialogue both patient and nurse are calling and responding all at once. The patient's request, for instance, is a call for help and at the same time a response to the nurse's availability or offer to be of help. From the other side, the *way* a nurse responds to a patient's call is, *itself*, a call to him for a particular kind of response, a call for his participation in the dialogue.

Reflect for a moment on your own example. Was your response to the patient influenced by the value you placed on such factors as his independence, motivation, rehabilitation, growth, strengths, pathology; on time, on place; on agency policy? Here again goal-directedness affects nursing dialogue. Our interpretation of the patient's calls as well as our responses are colored by the aim of our practice. Our values are like calls within the calls. Or to state it differently, the values underlying our practice give meaning to the calls.

Viewing dialogical nursing as a particular form of call and response highlights its complexity. It reveals the intricacy not only of its patterns of flow but also of its means of expression. Nursing is a lived call and response reflective of every mode of human communication.

Much has been studied and written about verbal dialogue between patient and nurse. Examining verbal exchanges from the perspective of call and response could uncover even more about this aspect of the nursing dialogue.

It is more difficult to find written descriptions of nonverbal nurse-patient communicaion, although this aspect is generally recognized to be of equal significance. Here again the call and response framework could be a useful aid. For instance, what does a nurse's mere physical presence mean to a patient either as a call or response? Or from the nurse's standpoint, under what circumstances is a patient's presence experienced as a call and, even more, as a call for a particular nursing response? What prompts us to respond in terms of his posture, his color, his facial expression, his behavior, the appearance of his clothes? Are we almost unconsciously checking some kind of "vital signs" in the intersubjective realm?

Nursing dialogue is characterized by the unique feature of occurring through nursing acts. The dialogue is experienced in what the nurse does with the patient. A call and response of caring is lived through in nurse-patient transactions (nursing care activities) from the simplest, most basic acts of bathing and feeding to the most dramatic resuscitation.

The nursing act itself contains a meaning for each person in the dialogue and the meanings may differ (for example, touching and being touched, feeding and being fed, bathing and being bathed). In addition, as a behavioral expression, the nursing act conveys a message, a reflection of the nurse's state of being (for example, anxious, hurried, troubled, absent, present, fully present). Furthermore, a nursing act may serve as an occasion, or even a catalyst, for opening or moving the dialogue in some direction on a verbal level (for example, bathing a patient may prompt his discussion of his body image or of his fear of disfigurement).

The complexity of possibilities in this unique feature of nursing dialogue (occurring through nursing acts) is staggering, expecially so when one considers the additional factors associated with the effects of technological advances in nursing. Think, for instance, of the influence on your nursing dialogue of any technical nursing procedure. What happens between you and the patient when you place a thermometer into his mouth? Take his blood pressure? Give him an injection? Aspirate him? Do any form of monitoring, from the simplest to the most complex? Are the technical procedures and instruments bridges or barriers in the between?

DIALOGICAL NURSING IN THE REAL WORLD

It is necessary now to look again at dialogical nursing in a broader perspective, for by limiting the exploration to the nurse, the patient, and their between, the previous discussion grossly oversimplified the way the dialogue actually evolves in real life. In the above, it was as if nursing were a drama acted out by two characters on a specially designed stage where precisely placed props lay ready to serve the actors and the passage of time is controlled by the chiming of a clock or the dimming of lights. As it is actually lived, the nursing dialogue is subjected to all the chaotic forces of real life. Nursing takes place in a real world of men and things in time and space. In many cases, it is a special world, a health system world, within the everyday world.

Other Human Beings

The dialogue lived between nurse and patient is affected by their numerous other interhuman relationships. For a nurse to be genuinely with a patient involves her coexperiencing his world with him. His family, friends, and significant others are a very real part of this world whether they are physically present or distant. So to be open to the patient is to be open to him as a person necessarily related to other men.

Futhermore, in caring for a patient the nurse relates to him not only as an individual patient but also as one in a group of patients. The group may be physically present (for example, in a ward, in an intensive care unit, in a waiting room, in a dining room, in a therapeutic group) or they may be present in the nurse's mind (for example, while caring for one she may think "I have three more patients to visit," "so and so needs his medication in five minutes," "I promised so and so I'd get back to him," "three other patients are waiting to be fed"). Even when the nurse is responsible for only one patient, she often views him in relation to other patients she has nursed.

The nurse herself also functions within complex networks of interhuman relationships that affect the nursing dialogue. As health care becomes more specialized, more groups of health care workers arise and the various groups become more diversified. So the nurse's intersubjective transactions with her patients occur within an intra- and interdisciplinary milieu of constantly changing personnel, functions, and roles. While her own role is expanding, extending, deepening, broadening, becoming more specialized, she must relate with others undergoing similar change. And here again, as with the patients so with her colleagues, the nurse is constantly faced with the possibility and necessity of relating to others in terms of their functions and as persons.

Finally, it should be recognized that while it is easy and common to think of "the nurse" as synonymous with the function "nursing," in real life the nurse is a human being necessarily related to others. She learns to focus on those present in her here and now work situation. But she too is her history and brings to her work world all that she is and all that she is not inlcuding her past experienced and future anticipated interhuman relationships. So each nurse affects her peopled nursing world and is affected by it in her own unique way.

From the other side, the patient also enters into the nursing dialogue with his various networks of interhuman relationships. How he experiences his relationships with his family and significant others, with the patient groups of which he becomes a part in different degrees, with members of various disciplines and health services groups, with "the" nurse and "his" nurse, all influence the lived nursing dialogue. It is always colored by the patient's current mode of interpersonal relating. Of course, the current mode reflects his past, for example, learned habits of response, and his future, for example, concerns about anticipated changes in interpersonal relationships due to the effects of his illness. In some cases, the intersubjective behavior itself becomes the focus of the nursing dialogue as the area of the patient's greatest needs in attaining well-being and more-being.

Things

The nursing dialogue takes place in a real world of things, ordinary things of everyday living and all forms of health care equipment. Both types of objects affect the nurse-patient transactions and their influence varies for they may be experienced differently by nurse and patient.

Ordinary objects used everyday—eating utensils, clothes, furniture, books, television sets—are so familiar that one usually takes their use for granted.

However due to illness a person may be unable to manipulate a knife and fork, for example. They become frustrating objects. His tools are no longer extensions of himself but impediments and barriers. He feels handicapped. His world of things changes.

On entering a health care facility, the patient finds himself in a foreign world of strange objects. In place of his familiar possessions he is surrounded by equipment, machines, instruments, solutions, and so forth. He may experience these as bewildering, frightening, painful, supportive, soothing, life-sustaining. The nurse, on the other hand, may experience these same objects quite differently. To her they may be familiar tools, useful aids, complex machines, annoyingly defective equipment. Even in a situation that does not have special equipment, for instance in a home, the patient's world of things changes as the nurse converts ordinary objects into tools. Thus, while nurse and patient share a situation, the things in their shared world have different meanings for each. The things themselves as well as the persons' relations to them can serve to enhance or inhibit the intersubjective transaction of nursing.

Time

To view dialogical nursing as it is actually experienced in the real world, one must conceive of it as occurring in time, not simply measured time but also time as lived by patient and nurse. Certainly both participants are caught up in measured time and this influences their shared world, for example, eight-hour tours of duty, a day off, surgery scheduled at 8:00 a.m., discharge in two days, visit three times a week, clinic appointment in 30 days. Thus, to an extent, both patient and nurse must live by the clock and calendar.

However, equally important, or perhaps even more important, in the lived dialogue of nursing is the participants' experience of time. Some references were made to lived time in the section on call and response where it was noted how the nursing dialogue unfolds over time from moments to years. How the involved persons experience this continuity is an individual matter.

The nurse may conceive of herself as one of many persons contributing to a continuous stream of caring for the patient. So she will give and hear and write and read reports, note observations, keep records. She will carry an image of the patient in her mind continually adding to it or changing it with each interaction or report. Sometimes, after not seeing the patient for a time, on meeting him again she will "pick up where she left off," treating him as if he were the same person, as if days, months, years of living had not intervened. "Oh, it's him again." Or she may be startled by the visible changes and resume the dialogue from that point. Or even if change is not visible, she may be aware that it may have occured and try to fill in the gap.

These possiblities may be mirrored from the patient's standpoint, for he likewise experiences continuity or lack of it in his care. And yet, the experience must be different for him. For instance, nurses may think of continuity of care in terms of "coverage" for a planned program of care. So it has often been claimed that "the nurse is with the patient 24 hours a day." From the patient's point of view this is not true. *A* nurse may be with him but each nurse is different. The function of nursing may be continuous, but individual nurses come and go; the day nurse, the evening nurse, the night nurse are each unique individuals. And the nursing dialogue as lived, intersubjective transaction occurs between a particular nurse and a particular patient.

When we speak of a nurse and a hospitalized patient spending a day together, we usually are referring to eight hours out of a 24-hour day. They may both experience the spacing of this time by functions or activities such as meal time, medicine time, visiting time. Yet the measured minutes and hours are experienced differently by each in their different modes of being in the situation. Nurses often express feelings of not having enough time to give the care they want to give; of having too many demands on their time; of trying to "make time" for patients who ask "do you have a minute?" Patients live their time in relation to boredom, pain, loneliness, separation, waiting. The nursing dialogue runs its course in clock time but both nurse and patient live it in their private times.

When the nursing dialogue is genuinely intersubjective, it has a kind of *synchronicity* that is evident in the nurse's being with and doing with the patient. This kind of timing is related to the transactional character of nursing and to its goal of nurturing the development of human potential. It is experienced in openness, availability, and presence, as well as in nursing care activities. The nurse feels in harmony with the rhythm of the dialogue and, sensing the timing of its flow, she paces her call and response to patient's ability to call and respond in that moment. So, as a nurse, you may find yourself almost unconsciously or intuitively waiting, holding back, anticipating, urging the patient. This kind of synchronization or timing is intersubjective for the clues or reasons for encouraging or waiting are not found solely in the patient's behavior nor only in the nurse's knowledge or experience. "Good" or "right" timing somehow involves the "between." It implies that nurse and patient share not only clock time but private, lived time.

Space

By exploring the dialogue of nursing as it is lived in the real world the factor of space becomes apparent. Here again the dialogue is influenced by space as it is measured and space as it is experienced by nurse and patient. When thinking of health care facilities, "space" may be synonymous with such things as beds, waiting rooms, interview rooms, treatment areas, size of patient's room, visiting areas, a quiet place, a private place. Naturally, the physical setting, whether in a hospital, home, anywhere in the community, can serve to enhance or impede the nursing dialogue. However, the person's experience of the space may be even more important.

Space is lived in terms of large and small, far and near, long and short, high and deep, above and below, before and behind, left and right, across, all around, empty, crowded. These perceptions and experiences of space may be influenced by the effects of illness, for example, changes in vision or locomotor ability. Thus, a patient's spatial world may change, expand or diminish, become unmanageable or manageable day by day. Furthermore, a patient's attitude toward and experience of a particular place may be affected by his mental association to it (for example, oncology ward, psychiatric unit), his previous experience in it (for example, emergency room, operating room), or a desire to be somewhere else (for example, "This is a nice hospital but I'd rather be home").

Place is a kind of lived space. It is personalized space. One says, for example, "Come to my place" meaning to my home. Or even more personally, it relates to where I feel I belong or am, for instance, "he put me in my place; I felt put down." The patient may feel "out of place" in the health care setting, while it may be commonplace to the nurse. There may be areas in the setting that the patient experiences as his territory, for example, his bed, his room, his ward; while other areas are "theirs" or "restricted to authorized personnel." So a nurse and a patient may be in a place together, yet one feels at home and the other does not. For the nurse to be really *with* the patient involves her knowing him in *his* lived space, in his here and now.

Lived space is interrelated with lived time. Patients hospitalized for a long time often express a proprietary attitude toward the hospital. The same holds true for personnel. With time and familiarity a feeling of reciprocal belongingness grows. The person belongs in the place and the place belongs to the person. On the other hand, when a person finds himself in a new place he may feel the discomfort of not belonging. This is as true for the nurse in an unfamiliar setting as for the patient. Again in this regard, the lived nursing dialogue is enhanced by the nurse's awareness of not only her own experience of space but the patient's as well.

CONCLUSION

This chapter explored the basic view of humanistic nursing as a phenomenon in which human persons meet in a nurturing, intersubjective transaction. Beginning with the central intuition that nursing is lived dialogue, the exmination turned to its existential source, the nursing situation as it is lived. Reflection on actual experience clarified the phenomena of meeting, relating, presence, and call and response as they occur in humanistic nursing. Dialogical nursing was then reconsidered in broader perspective as it actually evolves in the real world of men and things in time and space.

As scientific advances multiply in the health field, nursing is swept along in the tide. Continuous technological changes, ever increasing specialization, emphasis in nursing education and research on scientific methodology all have marked influence on the development of nursing. Science (with a capital S) colors the nursing world. At every turn it permeates the nurse's being with and doing with the patient. It offers a certain security by providing a consistent and effective approach to some problems and questions, and, in some cases, results in general laws to guide practice. At the same time, in the lived nursing world the nurse experiences a reality that is not open to the scientific approach, a reality not always verifiable through sense perception, a reality of individuality. The uniqueness of individuality (her own as well as the patient's) pervades the nursing dialogue.

The ever-present individual differences may be regarded as intractable elements to be conquered for the sake of the efficiency of the system (for example, fit the patient to the treatment program). Or they may be valued as indicators of the inexhaustible richness of human potential to be developed. In their daily practice, nurses are drawn toward the two realities—the reality of the "objective" scientific world and the reality of the "subjective-objective" lived world. This tension is lived out in the nursing act. Doing with and being with the patient calls for a complementary synthesis by the nurse of these two forms of human dialogue, "I-It" and "I-Thou." Both are inherent in humanistic nursing for it is a dialogue lived in the objective and intersubjective realms of the real world.

In the highly complex health care system nurses experience many demands from many directions. Their clinical judgments in daily practice must be made within a continuous stream of decisions about priorities of investment of their time and efforts. Sometimes, survival in the system reduces the nurse to following the line of least resistance, that is, responding to the immediate or to the loudest demands. However, even with their total commitment this course of response does not guarantee that nurses are making their greatest possible contribution to health care. This can happen only if we are able to see demands and opportunities in relation to our reason for being—nurturing the well-being and more-being of persons in need.

Humanistic nursing, viewed as a lived dialogue, offers a frame of orientation that places the center of our universe at the nurse-patient intersubjective transaction. Insightful recognition of the lived nursing act as the point around which all our functions revolve, could require a Copernican revolution of orientation of some nurses. It does provide, for all nurses, a true sense of direction that can be actualized by each unique nurse through creative human dialogue.

4

PHENOMENON OF COMMUNITY

Humanistic nursing creates, happens within, and is affected by community. This chapter will discuss the abstract term "community." To stimulate thought on a nurse's influence on community, consideration will be given to three points: (1) my angular view of community and its evolvement, (2) how man has considered community over time, (3) how a human being comes to be through community.

MY ANGULAR VIEW

One can view members of a family, a student class, a hospital unit, a hospital staff, several related hospital staffs, health services organizations within a geographic area, a profession, a town to a world or universe as community. Man's mind, my mind, determines where I superimpose the limits or lift the limits or relate components. In *The Republic* Plato depicted a community as a macrocosm.[1] Its nature was conditioned by the kinds of men, the microcosms, that composed it. The macrocosm was a reflection of its microcosms.

So each human person, each nurse, as a microcosm, could make a difference. Reflecting on the lived worlds of nurses, their communities, if we use Plato's philosophical analogy of macrocosm-microcosm, despite the varieties of situation, we can make meaningful a basic concept of community. Such a concept utilized by a nurse to view her particular ongoing changing world can help her to understand more realistically, survive within, and strugglingly participate as a quality force.

To be a quality force within community a nurse must open her being to the endless innovative possibilities and unattempted choices available to her.

---

[1] Plato, *The Republic*, trans. Francis MacDonald Cornford (New York: Oxford University Press, 1945).

The ability to thus open one's self requires our exposing our biases, the shades through which we regard the world, to the sunlight. In nursing our shades often are closed categories, labels, diagnoses, trite superficial hackneyed expressions learned by us, taught to us as fact, taken in unexamined, and left unreexamined despite other changes in ourselves and our situations. Socrates said, and it still holds, that the unexamined life is not worth living. Our shades can be cherished concepts, beliefs that guide us automatically rather than thoughtfully. Whether they are entirely myth or partial truths, they can cause us agonizing dilemma because they obscure the obviously relevant and the possibilities beyond. A concept of community, if grasped and if a nurse is truly consciously aware, can help her to understand how her nursing world has evolved, is presently, and how she can be, to shape its future in accordance with her values.

As nurses one of our shades is often the confining labels we give to ourselves as doers in service giving profession. I would like to go on record as most respectful of this aspect of my world. I regret, nonetheless, that we have not always similarly crystallized and floodlighted the discovery and creative possibilities in our communities. In our very personal, intimate, involved professional nursing relations with other man we are privileged to be included in human happenings open to no other group. As nurses, we have had and are having emphasized to us the importance of facts handed to us. Can we actuate the importance of the knowledge of man that becomes part of us through our nursing worlds? It is hard to honor the significance of the everyday, the commonplace, the intimately known? It has been said that one could know of the whole universe if one could make every possible relationship starting from a piece of bread. Think of a "simple" or "routine" nursing situation. Think of its true complexity and how it can trigger puzzlement, wonderment, and thinking. As learning situations, nurses' situations are existentially priceless. Returning now to Plato's conception of community understood through the terms macrocosm and microcosm, what can the nursing world situation reveal to us of community? What are the qualities of the participants, the microcosms, and how are these qualities reflected in our nursing communities?

HISTORY: THE SHADES OF MY WORLD, BRACKETED

In years past as a public health mental health psychiatric nurse I have structured facts about man, family, and community precisely for presentation. Approaching the data sociopsychologically I framed it in the public health model of promotion of health, prevention of illness, treatment, rehabilitation, and maintenance. I thought of family sociologically as nuclear, procreative, and extended. In accordance with the psychoanalytic model, family members were oral, anal, oedipal, latent, homosexual, adolescent, heterosexual, and/or mature. Community, like person and family, was considered according to a closed paradigm, ranging from ideal to abysmal, from the smallest to the largest unit in which persons congregated for common purposes. I selected from experience nursing examples to make these sociopsychological public health constructs meaningful. I did not start from nursing experiences to come up with nursing concepts of man, family, and community. I denied my particular self as a source of knowledge of these areas. Had education programmed me to value only others' ideas gleaned in the classroom or from books? I projected this devaluation of my own ideas onto my colleagues and until I really knew them gave them what I thought they wanted, others' ideas. Presently I prize my uncertainty about the nature of man in family and community and my striving toward an ever explorative process of being and becoming, available for surprise. Paradoxically, I believe it was these very same capacities, uncertainty and striving, that compelled my superimposing on my colleagues with certainty other persons' and other professions' views. Actually, my certainty about the conundrums: man, family, community come only in particulars and only in fits and starts, and my certainty is at once a truth and a nontruth. I see my aim as ever striving toward certainty while constantly wrestling with the discomfort of uncertainty.

EACH NURSE: A *NOETIC LOCUS*[2]

Each nurse is a "knowing place." It feels as if my greatest talents, as a human nurse person, awaited my acceptance that came through as I related to the existentialist thinking of persons like Martin Buber, Teilhard de Chardin, Frederick Nietzsche, Karl Popper, Hermann Hesse, Wilfrid Desan, and Norman Cousins. Now when I think of the phenomena—man, family, community—Theresa G. Muller, nurse educator and clinician, who quoted Hersey from his novel, *A Single Pebble*, comes to mind.[3] He said, "I approached the river as a dry scientific problem; I found it instead an avenue along which human beings moved whom I had not the insight, even though I had the vocabulary, to understand." I consider my greatest gifts as a human being nurse my ability to relate to other man, to wonder, search, and imagine about my experience, and to create out of what I come to know. My ever developing internalized community of world thinkers dynamically interrelated with my conscious awareness of my experienced nursing realm allows my appreciation of my human gifts and the ever enrichment of myself as a "knowing place."

NURSE: EXPERIENCE INTERNALIZED

Nursing experience taught me that each man, each family, each community was at once alike and different. Hesse, an existential novelist, in *Steppenwolf*,

---

[2] Wilfrid Desan, *Planetary Man* (New York: The Macmillan Company, 1972).
[3] John Hersey, *A Single Pebble* (New York: Alfred A. Knopf, 1956), p. 18.

describes each man who has become in family and community as like an onion with hundreds of integuments or a texture with many threads.[4] Then man's differences would be in the quality of his integuments and their development or in his threads in their preponderance. Contemplating the struggles in community regarding mutual understanding, I expanded Hesse's conception of man and found my vision of community to be a salad tossing or a patchwork quilt tumble drying.

Valuing the complexity of this conception of man and therefore of community I find myself smiling at the naivety of the earlier more static frames of order I superimposed on these phenomena. These oversimplifications maintained the shade through which I viewed my world. The shade was: others are knowing places, they are responsible; therefore if I quote authority from outside of myself, I can speak with certainty about what I know and believe and no one can attack me. And yet, my unique knowledge was not given and so my defense, my clutching at security foiled my human need for conceptualization of and expression of my own nurse vision of reality. This defeated the development by me of nursing theory.

Now I realize how I underestimated the potentialities of my nursing effect, of the difference I made, and could make. Just consider the given human uniqueness of each participant in the nursing situation whose familial potential goes back to an origin of thinking being or consciousness, and forward to his anticipation of the future, his eternity.

In the nursing literature, it is rather infrequent that we philosophically share our innermost thoughts, dreams, ideals, and strivings without a strong overlay of indoctrination or conversion. Nietzsche presents philosophy as autobiographical, such sharing does not offer maps. It could offer relevant resources and stimulate other nurses to influence the shape and becoming of the profession.

This chapter attempts to discuss ideas of community, the macrocosm, by considering man, the microcosm, as he develops in family and community. The ideas represent my "here and now" as it reflects my past and anticipated nursing world, including my hopes and expectations.

Man's Experience

Each human being carries a view of persons, families, and communities shaded by the views of his nuclear family. The past usually is corrected; it is never erased. So in his family of origin man internalizes ideas of "right-wrong," "appropriate–inappropriate," "expected–unexpected." Each family's shaded world echos its procreators' familial, psychosocialeconomic, religious and experiential breadth, closely resembled or distorted. Two persons, perhaps more, usually husband and wife, bring shaded views together in some combination or balance that becomes the "stuff," the authority, of

[4] Hermann Hesse, *Steppenwolf* (New York: Holt, Rinehart and Winston, 1966), p. 60.

their childrens' worlds. Thus, children see their early worlds through the complementariness and conflict of this intial home view, acting at times with it; at times against it.

Adults, in response to and through one another, procreate new sensitive beings whom they want and/or do not want and whom they may and/or may not experience as their responsibility in varying degrees. Marcel, a French existentialist philosopher, views procreation and responsible parenthood as quite different. My past nursing experience substantiates this. Marcel expresses my bias about responsible parenthood, and this statement is also worthy of consideration by nurses in positions of authority to others. He says, "We have to lay down the principle that our children (or those for whom we care) are destined, as we are ourselves, to render a special service, to share in a work, we have humbly to acknowledge that we cannot conceive of this work in its entirety and that *a fortiori* we are incapable of knowing or imagining how it is destined to shape itself for the young will, it is our province to awaken to a consciousness of itself.[5] Think of this statement of responsible authority. How has it been evidenced in families and nursing situations of your nursing world? What are your expectations of your patients or nurses with whom you work?

Teilhard de Chardin, paleontologist, biologist, and philosopher, like Nietzsche, depicts man as lacking a fixed nature with his own mode of being as his fundamental project.[6] Initially, each person takes on a mode of being in his world dependent upon his degree of freedom and the how and what of the world as presented by his family and perceived by him. The world as presented is reflective of the family's culture, their provincial world view, their unique experienced "here and now," and the times. Metaphorically, the family's lived world, how they experience at this particular cross-section of their lives, can be symbolically described as a kaleidoscopic telescoping of its past and anticipated future. Now, this would be what was presented at any particular time. What would a child's perception do to this metaphorical symbol? The child's current human development and his narrow experience would be like a circus house mirror that would interpret the metaphorical symbol distortedly. Witness a three-year-old speaking questioningly and complainingly about her tension headache to her mute, nonperceptive doll, and asking her to please, please stop making such a mess and racket.

The earliest childhood views of family and community are influenced over time, gradually and abruptly, and grow in complexity. The child's puzzlement is aroused by others' comings and goings, happenings within the family, immediate neighborhood, and adjacent community, and the world presented through books and technologically, on radio, television, and tape recorder. Each child attends these presentations with varying measures of complacency, questioning, bafflement, and involvement.

---

[5] Gabriel Marcel, *Homo Viator* (New York: Harper & Row, Publishers, Harper Torchbooks, 1962), p. 121.

[6] Teilhard de Chardin, *The Phenomenon of Man* (New York: Harper & Row, Publishers, 1961).

For instance, for myself, as a child there was the excitement of the construction of a new house in the woods next door and meeting new neighbors. Initially my parents expressed their differences from ourselves. The differences they perceived were followed by negative projections on these unknown folk. Were these others really humanly different? I investigated; my family investigated. The folk became persons. They expressed themselves differently in volume and sometimes in language. They looked different. Yet they were not fearsome. They felt, cared, responded, and worried much as we did. Mutual knowledge allowed increasing closeness and liking.

Forbidden! This was the neighborhood across the tracks. I cried when an uncle teasingly proclaimed one day that my missing mother was over there. Later I attended school with both white and black children who lived over there. And again, each was different, yet not different; each was knowable, likeable, and loveable.

Adult family members whispered about a neighbor woman from across the street. She was apparently hospitalized permanently. When I inquired as to why, eyebrows were raised and strange looks were exchanged. I was told in a not believable way, "She broke her leg falling off the back porch."

A neighbor husband and wife frequently could be heard fighting both verbally and physically. Family talk at our house depicted the husband as "evil," the wife as a "poor soul." I did not enjoy being in these peoples' house. Perhaps the violence frightened me; perhaps I was uncertain when it might errupt? Perhaps I was concerned that I might one day somehow become part of such a situation? Now, looking back over the years, I would guess that both this husband and wife were "poor souls" struggling with their humanness as best they could.

An adolescent girl lived down the block. She was labeled as "strange," "peculiar," "odd," "crazy." Ofen one saw her talking to herself, skipping and rotating as she moved along in her always solitary and mysterious way. All expressed great sorrow for her always solitary and mysterious way. All expressed great sorrow for her elderly mother and father on her admission to the "State Hospital." Years later I wondered, and still wonder what happened to that girl, herself? What kind of an existence has she experienced?

During these early years there was also separation from and loss of close loved family members. When I was three and a half a great aunt who always appreciated my side of things moved out of our home due to a family argument. Perhaps most confusing of all during these preschool years, at four and a half, my father died suddenly. "They" said that he went to heaven, that God called him. Why did he go? Why would he leave us? Most important how could he leave me? What had I done wrong? Was it that I had not loved him enough? Been good enough to him? Was he angry? What kind of God is God, anyway? Is he benevolent, malevolent, indifferent? Is he real: is he believable? What can one expect and how should one act toward authority and power? The world didn't feel like a very safe place nor did persons appear to be dependable.

Then there was school. With additional authorities and peers there arose new wonderment and expectation. The way one was to be in school was different from at home. And what was happening at home while I was at school? Could I depend on things being safe? In kindergarten I made an ash tray of clay for my already dead father.

In my child world there were books, radio, and the movies. Today children experience these, as well as television and record players. For me, books, radio, and the movies brought into my world new aspects of fear, excitement, joy, love, horror, violence, imagination, and suspense. They depicted at times the ideal and at times the abysmal. Sometimes, despite everything, good triumphed. At other times regardless of the effort invested all was lost. Where was the harmony of logical reason? Is our world absurd? Are we absurd to respond to it with an expectation of reason?

For each child there are very special, long-rememberd events: being taught to swim by one's father, family picnics, trips into the world beyond city or country, going to the circus, a world's fair, a zoo or a fantasy land. There, also are the events of being loved and loving deeply, linked somehow with times of of feeling unloved and unloving.

More than earlier, today there multiple community groups for children where activities are guided and supervised. Within these situations and in the free play of neighborhood children, there is always the confusing, enlightening, and frequently distorted information gained through discovering your relationship with both boys and girls. Exploration by children into their sexual similarities and differences, a healthy pursuit, in the past more than today often aroused parental furor. Furor and different reactions from different involved parents lead to further child confusion and focus.

Within childhood peer relations there are games, play, and schoolwork that allow the child to come to know personally the meanings and feelings of competing, collaborating, fighting, winning, losing, destroying, building, aggression, passivity, constriction, freedom, and choice.

Then there is adolescence with all its moodiness, questions, fears, and experimenting related to adult modes of being. The moods are a mystery and the questions often unanswerable or the answers contradictory. Norman Kiell in *The Universal Experience of Adolescence* says that as adults we forget the intensity, turmoil, and concretes of this period and that perhaps we have to.[7] Yet, it is not possible that the instability and discomfort of spirit lived in adolescence does not leave its ingrained tracing as part of our eternal presents.

When the focus of our responsibility shifts from play to work, during these early years of becoming, depends on our particular circumstances and abilities. For most persons there is a tipping of the balance between these. Hopefully neither extreme is the master. Fortunately, in many instances, as the child's work as been to play; the adult's work world, his world of responsibility is lived, experienced by him, to an extent as play—it give satisfaction and pleasure.

---

[7] Norman Kiell, *The Universal Experience of Adolescence* (New York: International Universities Press, 1964), pp. 22-44.

Some adults select another and are chosen by this other for a sharing of their worlds. Some go it alone. Some procreate new beings; some create in other ways; some give-take and exist; some just lean. These last appear to be, and yet to not be, "all-at-once."

MAN BECOMES EVER MORE

Buber perceives man becoming more through his human capacity to relate to other being in all forms from the materialistic to the spiritual in "I-Thou," "I-It," and "We" ways.[8] Gestation, with the closeness of mother and child, has left man with an ingrained knowing of the experience of closeness. Thus, throughout man's life his condition of existence is affected by and desires relationship with and closeness to other being. The closeness of the conditions of gestation is never again possible, hence existential loneliness. Yet because of this prenatal experience Buber conceives of man as born with a "Thou"—another—before he is conscious of himself, his "I." With growing consciousness he sorts out his "I" from his "Thou." You can see the late infant doing, acting through, this separation. During this growing phase, often to the care-taking adult's frustration, he repeatedly, intensely, and excitedly throws his toys or bottle out of the crib, carriage, or playpen. Often he runs away from his "Thou," his parental security source, to a safe distance with intense awareness of what he is doing. While internalizing these and subsequent "Thous" as part of his "I," his knowing place, paradoxically, he sorts out who he is, and who and what is other than himself. So with ever more relationship, ever more experience, he becomes ever more the person he has the human capacity to be. He becomes more through his relations with others, never the same as these others, though he does internalize these others as part of himself.

Buber describes "I-Thou" relating, man merging with otherness, as always necessitating an "I," a man, capable of recognizing self as at a distance, apart from otherness. Therefore, his "I-Thou" relating, a merging of beings, is not like the psychological defense, unconscious identification. Buber's "I-Thou" relating emphasizes awareness of each being's uniqueness without a superimposing, or a deciding about the other without a knowing. Such relating is a turning to the other, offering the other authentic presence, allowing the authentic presence of the other with the self, and maintaining one's capacity to question. It is not then identification or an idealization of the other. Within this mysterious happening of "I-Thou" relating, when both participants are human, each becomes more. Buber refers to the event of this merging of other ness, of man with other being, as "the between." Humanistic nursing is concerned with "the between" of nurses and their others. Their others, the

---

[8] Martin Buber, *I and Thou,* 2nd ed., trans. Ronald Gregor Smith (New York: Charles Scribner's Sons, 1958).

microcosms of their communities, would be patients, patients' families, professional colleagues, and other health service personnel.

Buber describes man's ability to come to know and relate in "I-It" as man looking back, reflecting on his past "I-Thou" relations. Looking back these "I-Thou" relations are viewed as an object to be known, as "It". "I-It" relating allows man to interpret, categorize, and accrue scientific knowledge.

Finally man relates with others as "We." This permits the phenomenon of community and of adult unique contribution. So man becomes through relating with family, others, and community, like Hesse's onion or a being who actively moves toward ever more integuments, qualities, threads, and complexity.[9] Many unique contradictory type beings, then, have influenced the becoming of each individual human person. In a sense each unique person might be viewed as a community of the beings with whom he has meaningfully related in struggle and/or complementariness. In fact Buber talks of thinking man as a dialogue of internalized "Thous."

COMMUNITY: NURSING

If each man can be likened to a community of his internalized "Thous," logically think of the outcome of many men struggling together supposedly for a common purpose. Since time began, man in community has been experienced by man as chaotic. Thus Plato wrote *The Republic*.[10] This presentation depicted an impossible scheme for developing an ideal community. As a classic, *The Republic* continues to be a thought provoking thesis. Its antiquity makes one realize that this desire to control, our continued concern with genetic planning, is a part of the very nature of man. And yet, considering man's ever existing recognition of the chaos of community how naive we often behave, for example, enraged at experiencing *another* communication break.

Plato envisioned regulating and controlling almost every dimension of the individual's existence in accordance with his particular potential for development to fulfill the needs of his ideally conceptualized community. Today Heinlein, a science fiction novelist, still writes of breeding for longevity in man, as we breed animal stock for the greatest amount of meat and profit.[11] Giving Plato his due, he recognized at the end of his book concern and doubt as to whether men so carefully mated and reared would fulfill their designated responsibilities. He wondered if things could, would, or would not go in accordance with his plan. He then logically indicated the process and kinds of community deteriorations which could ensue. Plato had a concept of an ideal community, of ideal types of necessary men, and of ideal male–female breeding relationships. He viewed our present-style family as one that saps the

---

[9] Hesse, *Steppenwolf*, p. 60.

[10] Plato, *The Republic*.

[11] Robert A. Heinlein, *Time Enough for Love* (New York: G.P. Putnam's Sons. 1973).

strength of community and does not support this concept. He conceived of communal living more like the communal living of our present-day communes. However, Plato's communes would have been regulated by the plan as he conceived it. Existence in these communes was to be predetermined and very determined.

Nursing, though not generally the ruling force of this type of planning, certainly is involved in control measures analogous to Plato's. Nurses do influence who gets the hospital bed and who does not, who gets the specialized treatment and equipment, who is discharged and when, and what goes into the education and planning for post-hospital health care. Also, how do our biases influence our teaching regarding family? Innuendoes are frequent in the areas of birth control, abortion, and family size. So nurses can make a difference regarding community thought, purpose, and action.

Nietzsche put forth a concept of community of a more indefinite nature than Plato's.[12] Two major themes dominated the nature of community in his conception: (1) the legitimate purpose of community was the total support of its elite men and (2) the criterion for determining the elite was to be based on those who selected their own values with a "will" to say, "yes" to life. He referred to his elite as supermen. He questioned the realization of such a community because of the preponderance of conforming nonquestioning mediocre men. This complacent majority fearful of the different or strange would subdue the possibility of his supermen. Nietzsche did not seem to trust man; he spoke of him as "human, all too human." Unlike Plato, Nietzsche viewed "good" and "evil" as arising from a common source. Man in his humanness, Nietzsche felt, denied his animal heritage and animal qualities. Recognition of these, of one's Dionysian nature, as a source of both "good" and "evil" was necessary for becoming superman.

To me it is wondrous to ponder my own conscious purposefulness and unconscious purposelessness, my quality of force as a member of the nursing and health communities, viewed through the deep extensive conceptualized thought Nietzsche bequeathed. I offhand consider our communities as egalitarian, part of a larger egalitarian society. Are they really? Does the citizen affect the quality of organizational structure in accordance with his existential needs while in our commonplace—the health-nursing world? Whose values set and direct on this stage of life? Do I, nurse, search out the values on which I want to base my nursing practice? Do I look for direction and values from others? Did I take on values during my initial nursing experience—values never to be reexamined?

Within the nursing community are there nurses eagerly noncomplacent and desirous of looking at, of sharing their explorations, and of determining and choosing the values that they want to underlie their nursing practice?

---

[12] Frederich Nietzsche, "Beyond Good and Evil," trans. Helen Zimmern, in *The Philosophy of Nietzsche* (New York: Random House, 1927) and "Thus Spoke Zarathustra." trans. Thomas Common, in *the Philosophy of Nietzsche* (New York: Random House, 1927).

Would supernurses be allowed to be the mediocre many? Who would determine the elite of the nursing community? Could supernurses survive without approval of their being different? Would they be strengthened by the fruits of suffering in their struggle within the profession? Would these fruits of suffering contribute constructively to the strengthening of the nursing community?

Buber, like Nietzsche, sees man-in-community with possibilities for evolving, being, and becoming more. Buber trusts each man as a unique potential involved in an ongoing struggle with his fellows directed toward a center.[13] His nonstatic, nonselected community where men become in and through ongoing struggle with each other expresses the reality of my nursing world. Who would expect a community without struggle if they accepted each man as his history inclusive of antecedents that go back to beginnings of man's consciousness and of anticipations that go forth into this man's notions of eternity? Considering the complexity of each man's being and becoming, it is surprising that we come to understand each other in community at all, rather than the reverse.

How can we hope for a sustained thereness, presences of nurses with other man (patients, patients' families, professional colleagues, and other health service personnel) as "We" in an ongoing struggle of community considering their multitudinous differences? Norman Cousins, in *Who Speaks for Man,* comments on man's inability to respond affirmatively to those he experiences as different from himself.[14] For the human community to progress he suggests federation. A unity in which differences would be valued as promoting thought, human evolvement, and community advancement. Cousins gives examples of man's inhumanity to man based on differences viewed as nonvalues. The prevalence of this latter view of differences is very evident in our commonplace health-nursing world. Can nurses and other health care maintainers look at the ways they respond to differences consciously, and can they deliberately choose to be open to responding to them as valuable? Can we conceive of there being value in that which we see as "not right," "untrue," "wrong?"

The ability to be there, to stay involved in community with my fellows, is a problem worthy of concern to me as a nurse. How do I stay in an existential way with my contemporaires, patients, patients' families when their values in reality are so different from my own? How do I go beyond a negative judgmental to a prizing attitude that would open the possibility of seeing strengths in others' views perhaps lost, discarded, or never previously existent in my own? Nonsuperimposing of my own value system through recognizing and bracketing it is a difficult professional goal. And yet, a goal that if coupled with the courage for personal existence, could sustain me in the health-nursing community.

---

[13] Martin Buber, *Between Man and Man,* trans. Ronald Gregor Smith (Boston: Beacon Press, 1955).

[14] Norman Cousins, *Who Speaks for Man?* (New York: The Macmillan Company, 1953).

So for a health-nursing community to truly be actualized each nurse would prepare to be all it was possible for her to be as a nurse. Then, through exploration there would be a recognition of the reality of the existent community. Over time a merger of the values of the nurse and of the existing community would be reflected as moreness in each. The nurse would be more through her relation with the community; the community would be more through its relation with the nurse. Each would make an important difference in the other. The macrocosm, the community, would reflect the nurse's quality of presence. The microcosm, the nurse, would reflect the presence of the community with her. Each unique man becomes in community through communication with other uniquely different men.

Part 2

METHODOLOGY—A PROCESS OF BEING

5
TOWARD A RESPONSIBLE FREE RESEARCH NURSE IN THE HEALTH ARENA

ANGULAR VIEW

Research is an inherent component of humanistic nursing. What condition of humanness is necesssary in the nurse for the actualization of nursing's research potential? This chapter will attempt to share some brooding and mulling on this problem.

Nurses practice within ever-moving, changing settings where formulated plans frequently and suddenly go awry. Unexpected patient needs arise. Powerful others make both reasonbale and unreasonable demands. Depended on others fail us due to human frailty or lack of dependability. The nurse's setting, her researchable area, is the extreme opposite of her colleague's, the laboratory investigator's. Her area is beyond research control measures. Too, it lacks the quiet isolated atmosphere conducive to contemplation and creative thinking associated with research.

Conversely, it is oversaturated with the "stuff" of meaningful existence. It can stimulate questions to the frenzy of immobilization. The human nurse's system can become overloaded. Such overloading reflects the humanness of the nurse; like all man she can envision possibilities beyond any human being's ability of fulfillment.

Nurses know there are events in their commonplace worlds that scream for human interpretation, understanding, and attestation. The question becomes "how." This "how" depends on more than concretes and events in the nurse's setting. This "how" depends on relevant "ifs." The meaningfulness of the nursing world will be actualized conceptually "if" this is supported by institutional economic and administrative planners, other nurses, and intradisciplinary colleagues. For knowledge available and visible to nurses in the health setting to be preserved, conceptualized for durability, it needs to be valued by the institutional health community. Still, most necessary to its duration is the appreciating of this knowledge by the nurse, herself.

HUMAN CONDITION OF BEING: NURSE RESEARCHER

Initiation of a Nurse Researcher

The nurse student, recently arrived in her experiential world, is awed with the need to be cognizant of multitudinous factors. At this initial introductory phase one could say her "being" as a nurse is programmed or imprinted with: It is your responsibility to report and attend all the things that influence the response and comfort of those for whom you care. This programming supports and is supported by any already existing tendencies within the nurse student toward unrealistic, perfectionistic expectations of self.

Then in research courses, usually positivistically geared, her programming jams. Her system is fed: Select out, isolate, focus down on a single question, limit your variables, establish a protocol of operation, control for reliability and validity, tunnel your vision, and safeguard objectivity. The jamming is the result of the human nurse's capacity to see relationships between the part and the whole. Human intelligence, as a condition of humanness, demands this relating of one thing to another. Often such relating is intuitive, human, based on much thinking for purposes of understanding and solution. Yet, often it cannot be substanitated fully and conceptualized logically at specific times, therefore it is subjective.

To highlight the obvious in the above I attempted facetiousness. Many nurses acutely aware of the complexities, contradictions, and inconsistencies of their nursing worlds have struggled and used the positivistic method in research studies. Hence, they have isolated a researchable question, stated their basic assumptions, hypothesized outcomes, selected samples, established experimental and control groups, formulated methodologies, searched out and utilized appropriate findings, and have made recommendations. Usually these research efforts have advanced scientific knowing and knowledge of existents within the health–nursing situation. And yet, often these efforts have discouraged the research wonderment of the nurse interested in the nature and meaning of the nursing act and how the event of nursing is lived, experienced, and responded to by the participants. These positivistic research methods have made available answers. Still, they have not answered the questions most relevant to nursing practice and to nurses.

These nurses were certain that man generally could not be prescribed for interpersonally; he was not predictable, not yet an automaton. Faced with alternatives men often surprised. Consequently these positivistic approaches to studying human events, unless one forced one's data crowbar style, always terminated with a kind of miscellaneous category. Man's undeterminedness makes him all-at-once frustrating to study, impossible to distinctly categorize, and excitingly mysterious and the most worthy focus of nursing research.

A Nurse Researcher's Presence
in the Nursing—Health Setting

The existent, a nurse labeled researcher, in the health world brings a disquiet that has to be understood and endured. Necessities for scientific study in the nurse's world of the nursing event or situation are wonderment, concern, and responsibility. Open adherence to such qualities frequently startles others into speculating about the researcher. She, herself, becomes an oddity. Persons ponder the possibility of her study's having a hidden agenda that involves them. Over time these persons generally accept or reject the searcher's efforts. If rejected the searcher is often labeled a worthless nosey troublemaker. Subtly it is conveyed among those involved that she is to be interfered with often by mechanisms of ignoring or forgetting or righteously setting "patient's needs" above conforming to the study plan. For instance, how often have research nurses met with responses from staff at the time of their planned arrival on a unit to work with a patient, "Oh, he seemed to need activity, he was restless, I forgot you were coming, I sent him to the gym," or "Oh, (surprise) did you want to give the patient his morning care? That was done a while ago; we give care early." If accepted the searcher is often labeled an interested, interesting person whose efforts are to be fostered because her findings will enhance situation nursing. The distinction frequently is based in staffs' responses to the searcher's personality more than in the value of the issues of the investigation.

Significant to negative staff responses toward a nurse searcher is the necessity for her to withhold information. This withholding may be necessary to protect the study results. For example, it is necessary when a special type of patient care is being tested against usual patient care of when confidentiality is an issue. Confidentiality requires a nurse, searcher or not, to censor communications when personal knowledge of individuals make them identifiable. The need for confidentiality can be determined by the nurse's considering the knowledge gained in view of whether it will or will not influence the over-all treatment plan. If it will affect the plan, there is reason to reveal it; then it must be related in a manner that insures the patient's continued protection and, if possible, with his permission. If over-all treatment is not influenced, one must censor the knowledge gained to check one's own free communications. Would the patient want it revealed; is it knowledge of a quality that brings ridicule, is looked at negatively or nonacceptably in our particular culture generally? Is it of a sensitive nature and therefore knowledge we do not just reveal to anyone?

Other patient care givers may sense this withholding by the nurse searcher. They may reasonably accept it or unreasonably not accept it. The researcher may or may not be aware of or concern herself with her colleagues' sensitivity. This would depend on the searcher's usual modus operandi and on the importance she associates with her colleagues' sway in her investigation. The latter can be much greater than is obvious.

Confidentiality – Description:
Humanistic Nursing

Humanistic nursing practice theory proposes phenomenology, a descriptive approach to participants in the nursing situation as a method for studying, interpreting, and attesting the nature and meaning of the lived events. Humane nursing is not humanistic nursing within this theory unless that which becomes visible to the nurse in the nursing situation is shared in a durable form with colleagues.

Confidentiality, then, becomes an important issue in humanistic nursing. No scientific methodology of research is affixed with "ought" or "should" virtues regarding knowledge gained. In nursing, a professional helping realm, a practitioner or researcher is wed to "ought" and "should" virtues. The knowledge gained "ought" to be dispersed to colleagues for their increased understanding. It "should" enhance the constructive force of the profession. To so enhance it "must" be communicated in a manner that allows understanding while protecting distinct individuals and groups. Words and conceptualized ideas are the tools of phenomenology. Protection of distinct persons and meaningful communication can be augmented through the utilization of abstractions, metaphors, analogies, and parables. So humanistic nurses, as practitioners and researchers, are inherently responsible for their manner of being, responding, and consciously sculpturing knowledge into words.

Responsibility When Sharing:
Understanding of Man

How does a nurse searcher, who wonders, notices, relates, and comes to know, become humanly responsible? Nietzsche's philosophical works would direct a nurse searcher to look at her values. The values known through looking at what determines her actual behavior considering how these values correlate with her privilege of calling herself, nurse. Empathy, knowing how another experiences, when coupled with the title, nurse, dictates a performance that encompasses no harm to others and hopefully benefits them. Despite the human excitement of discovery, disciplined effort and rigorous evaluation enter into preparing knowledge of man for dispersal. Revelation should not merely shock; rather, professionally we use shock to awaken surprise, a fundamental, for human constructive movement toward moreness. The former, mere shock, needs to be guarded against. The latter, shock to awaken surprise needs to be exactingly, uncompromisingly attended for the communicability of knowledge and the actualization of the phenomenon, nursing.

In considering confidentiality and the quality of knowledge of man available to me, as nurse, my consciousness is confronted with my former mentor, and internalized "Thou," Paul V. Lemkau, M.D., psychiatrist. He emphasized repeatedly that the professional person, as he increasingly understands man, should take on increasing responsibility to man, one's self and one's others. Buber says, "As we become free. . . our responsibility must become personal and solitary."[1] One can extend this and say that to help others struggle for freedom one must realize that others must responsibly decide and that although they do this through and in the authentic presence of a nurse, these others are alone in deciding. And nurses in deciding what and how to convey of their knowing must decide freely, responsibly, personally, and alone.

The nurse in deciding what and how to convey, considering the professional necessities of both confidentiality and dispersion of knowledge, can be guided by a conception of the nature of man-in-his-world. Man in humanistic nursing practice theory is viewd as a conflictual, contradictory, inconsistent dilemma. One horn of the dilemma is ideal spirituality that wrestles against the other horn, protective materialistic animalism. This "all-at-once" struggling, stretched, mixed nature of man needs recognition. Recognition of man's nature, as such, supports greater self-acceptance. Self-acceptance and this view of man-in-his-world, like a magnifying glass, unmasks for a nurse her possible responses, motivations, and alternatives. Cognizant of these, she can responsibly select what knowledge to disperse to protect individuals and to continually shape and conceptually actualize the nursing profesion. Utilizing this magnifying glass on self in humanistic nursing practice theory to let one's existing mixed, varied, struggling reponses, motives, and alternatives into self-awareness is an axiom referred to as authenticity with self.

Acceptance of the others' human nature or human condition of being is usually easier than acceptance of our own. Usually each man is his own severest judge. Lilyan Weymouth, R.N., clinical specialist, my past teacher and present friend, in sympathetic moments, speaking of suffering others, often says, "the poor devils." Once, feeling anxious and annoyed, I responded, "we are all poor devils." She retorted, "I am glad you recognize that." Stopped short, I found myself continuing to ponder the phrase, "poor devils." Man's dilemma is that he is neither saint nor devil. He is a "poor saint" and a "poor devil," and by his nature he is pushed and pulled in both directions, "all-at-once." Our human existence in the world calls for an enduring with our virtues and vices, our energy and our laziness, our altruism and our selfishness, in a word with our humanness.

What meaning does this conception of man have for humanistic nursing practice theory? This theory necessitates a nurse who accepts and believes in the chaos of existence as lived and experienced by each man despite the shadows he casts interpreted as poise, control, order, and joy.

Labeled mental patients in therapeutic situation, in the sun beyond the shadows, express how they set themselves apart from the rest of the community

---

[1] Martin Buber, *Between Man and Man,* trans. Ronald Gregor Smith (Boston: Beacon Press, 1955), p. 93.

of man. They express how they experience themselves. They view themselves as the worst, the noblest, the unhappiest, the most maligned, and the most afraid. It comes out as if these superlative distinctions are their only claims to fame. In my humanness I appreciate the awesome dreads they live. They need to know that they exist in their unique distinctness. And yet, the separation and loneliness with which they adorn themselves and which professionally we have fostered with fear engendering diagnostic labels seem a heavier than necessary burden. In the light of existential loneliness, a part of each human existence, often I invite them to see themselves as not so unlike other men and as suffering the turmoil of existence as part of the human community, such as it is. One usually can note their surprise and disbelief of my view. Then, momentarily at least, tension seems to visibly fall from their faces and forms. When this idea of them is heard by them, its effect corresponds to how I experienced the technique in sensitivity group of literally being allowed to dance into what felt like the circle of man, our group.

To hear opportunities for humanistic nursing acceptance and support nurses, too, need to question their self-nurse-image within the nursing and health community. Do they know that they make and have real potential for making a difference, an important difference? Do they accept themselves as nurse? To me, a nurse is a being, becoming through intersubjectively calling and responding in her suffering, joyous, struggling, chaotic humanness, always trying beyond the possible while never completely free from ignoble personal human wants. And, through her presence it is possible for other persons to be all they can be in crisis situations of their worlds. For the nurse to be humanistic it is necessary for her to live her human condition-in-her-nursing-world proudly with all its vulnerability and all its wonders. As man, the nurse can recall and reflect on her "I," on her past "I-Other" experiences, and she can come to know and accept more and more of herself, as she becomes more. In humanistically recalling and reflecting a nurse will understand and respond empathetically and sympathetically to both her own humanness and the other's. She will recognize both self and other as "poor devil" and "poor saint," all-at-once.

On the other hand, if a nurse denies her own struggling humanness, she self-righteously will be apt to accuse either self or her other. This way of being denies, suppresses, and represses one's own and the other's ability to be, to be as much as potentially possible. Understanding man through this conception of him is important to the possibility of augmenting the implementation of humanistic nursing practice theory.

Authenticity With The Self:
For Actualization of Nursing's Potential

Husserl, the father of phenomenology, suggested the study of our lived worlds, our experience, a return to the study of "the thing itself." Looking at the lived worlds of nurses one is confronted with conflicts and multiple values. In their nursing worlds nurses often risk themselves in their commitment to good for their patients. They come to know aspects of their own and others' unique natures. These are often different from and frequently in conflict with generally accepted cultural values and/or institutional policies and rules. If confidentiality is an issue, does this dictate a suppression of nurses' complete knowing? Or does this call for a recognition of as complete a knowing as possible followed by responsible selection and revelation of that knowing which will advance knowledge and understanding of man? Understanding of man can change a person's way of being with other man and his way of existing in and responding to his world. I suggest the latter, as complete knowing as possible followed by responsible selection and revelation, with occasional risk taking to deepen the level of accepted cultural knowledge of man. Always, the nurse would protect an individual other man. This dispersion of knowlege, then, requires not only responsible being in the nursing situation but also mulling, pondering, assessing, and judging prior to disclosure.

As complete a knowing as possible, in humanistic nursing refers to its axiom, authenticity with the self. When I, nurse, respond in the arena of my lived nursing world, I respond to a particular person in this "here and now" with all my background and all my anticipation of the future. By respond, I do not mean to indicate that I overtly deliberately communicate or verbalize my total response. Rather I mean that I strive for *awareness* of my total response within myself to a particular person in a particular "here and now" viewed through my particular past and anticipated future. It is a struggle to grasp how I perceive and respond within all my capacity of human beingness. To attain the highest possible level of authenticity with the self requires later recollection of ongoing perceptions of the other and reciprocal responses, selected communications, and actions by the self. These recollections now become raw data available for analyzing, questioning, relating, synthesizing, hypothetically considering, and ongoing correcting. Sometimes sharing such recollections with a trustworthy confidant (clinical specialist, consultant) for purposes of reality testing is helpful. Often this can broaden the professional meaning base I attribute to both my perceptions and my responses. On return to the arena of my nursing world I then verify my perceptions. I can let the other know how I perceived his actions and be open to his further expression of how this world is for him. In professional nursing this kind of experiencing, searching, validating, utilizing of one's human potential capacity must be based in the ideals on which nursing rests. Primarily for me, I see myself, nurse, as comforter or being nurse in such a way that my other is helped to be all that he can humanly be in this particular "here and now" considering his unique potential.

So, being authentic with the self, is not an acting out of a nonthought through response or merely a doing of what one feels like doing. Rather it is the very opposite of this. It is a thought through responsible choosing of overt response based in knowledge and on nursing values. It must correspond positively with one's belief that searching and sharing in one's nursing world will promote both the nursed and the nurse to be more. If it is merely a peeking in on, an exploitation of the other, for selfish learning purposes, it desecrates the very concept of nursing. One has the broad human potential of feeling like doing many things, all-at-once, that extend into all kinds of living. And this is true in, as well as outside, a nurse world. In recollecting and reflecting on perceptions and responses in all these extremes one becomes freer to select from within one's self the values to be chosen, actualized, and potentiated in one's nursing practice. Authenticity with the self calls forth confrontation of the self with one's motivations and alternatives. This permits a purposeful selection and an aware actualized overt response based on one's nursing value criteria artfully tailored to a particular situation.

I consider each nurse a scientific-artist: classical, modern, primitive, cubic, or interpretive. My inference here is that we express artfully in accordance with our uniqueness. Many nurses given the same data would accomplish with the same or a similar degree of adequacy through use of their particular distinct selves. Therefore, though the function called for might be the same, each nurse would approach the function and the patient differently. How one actualizes the result of thinking, and being authentic with one's self recalls what Jung said about art.

> "Art is a kind of innate drive that seizes a human being and makes him its instrument. The artist is not a person endowed with free will that seeks his own ends, but one who allows art to realize its purpose through him. As a human being he may have moods and a will and personal aims, but as an artist he is "man" in a higher sense—he is "collective man"—one who carries and shapes the unconscious, psychic life of mankind."[2]

Through the years, over and over, I have met nurses so driven, motivated, and expressive in their nursing worlds.

I called this section "authenticity with the self: for actualization of nursing's potential." In it I have been trying to say, the more of ourselves we are able to awarely include, the more of the other we can be open to and with. A capacity for presence with others allows us to share ourselves. Through this sharing others become more. They are able to internalize us as "Thou." This happening occurs in the reverse, too, and we become more.

In a nursing situation the quality of being authentic with the self is to be striven for. It is a taking advantage of and appreciating of our human ability and spirit. It fosters our pursuit of inquiry, improves our caring for others, the contributing of our unique knowing, and it allows us to shape ever further a scientific-artistic profession of nursing.

Authenticity With the Self: Potentiated in Lived Experience

This example is offered to support the claims for authenticity with the self made in the last paragraph of the prior section.

---

[2] Carl G. Jung. *Modern Man in Search of a Soul,* trans. W.S. Dell and Cary F. Baynes (New York: Harcourt, Brace and World, 1933), p. 169.

As clincial supervisor and thesis advisor to a young graduate nursing student in her twenties the benefits of authenticity with the self were again brought home to me. She was taping her therapy sessions with two patients. These taped materials were to become her thesis data.

One of her patients was not much younger than herself. The other was a divorced woman in her forties, around my age. This young graduate nursing student was receiving clinical nursing supervision as a necessity in her particular situation not by personal choice or awareness of need.

From the onset of her clinical supervision with me I was aware that it aroused her feelings about dependence. At her age this had meaning since she was still struggling for independence and interdependence. This is a difficult time. Her response to me was "respectful," sweetly and unawarely hostile, and she made it apparent that I was another nurse authority to be appeased, manipulated, and outsmarted. This behavior had been successful for her with past authorities. She was bright and had been able to complete intellectual requests and assignments at the last minute with little effort. During the initial phase of our relationship awareness of her struggle, her difficulties and her assets, allowed me to maintain a supportive kind of being with her.

In listening to her therapy tapes I realized that another clinical supervisory approach was called for. She was defending against relating to her older patient by behaving toward her as she probably felt toward her own mother, and often toward me. Also, she was defeating her therapeutic purpose with her younger patient by viewing her as if the patient were herself. The older suicidal, depressed patient was begging her for an understanding therapeutic relationship. She needed terribly to share her suffering. This woman did not need a "rejecting daughter" working hard to outwit her. The younger patient needed to share her angry feelings and sense of worthlessness.

Through the tapes and through weekly sessions with the graduate student, I came to know and understand her existing nursing situations. At this time neither the student's need to understand nor the patients' theapeutic needs were being met. The student, too, was aware of this in a sort of suppressed way. Indirectly, in responding to her patients, knowing I would be listening to the tape she would take a "sweet swipe" at me which placed the responsibility of all our efforts on my shoulders. So if there were no beneficial outcomes, obviously the blame could be placed.

During the initial phase of my relationship with the graduate student and during the initial phases of her relationship with her patients I came to understand. I listened, got into the rhythm of these other spirits, reflected on what I had come to know, and out of this experience assessed and planned.

Later, taking what I had come to know, as just how it was for all of us, I shared my knowing with the graduate student and budding first-rate therapist. Together we explored the implications of the above. She became invested, involved, and excited about herself becoming more. We, myself and each of her patients, become for her more whom we essentially were. Most important to her and to me, this graduate student grew in her recognition and acceptance of herself and her ability as an adult nurse therapist. The thanks and meaningful praise she received from both her patients on termination of therapy made this apparent. It brought tears to both her eyes and mine. I felt joy in being with a now-respected colleague, as opposed to the earlier being with a person who felt like an unasked for "awe struck defensive daughter."

Authenticity with myself, and this graduate student's ability for authenticity with herself allowed these patients' progress to occur. It allowed a realistic articulation in this student's phenomenological master's thesis of her lived nurse experience. From such articulation will a theory and scientific-artistic profession of nursing ever mold, flow, and form.

WORDS DISTINCTLY HUMAN: LIMITING, YET HUMANIZING

Through words we humanly share the meaning to us of our behavior, experience, and profession. Words attest to and endure. Thus, a professional history is possible, accrues, and has lasting duration. The study of the nursing event itself and its conceptualization as proposed in humanistic nursing practice theory is an application of phenomenology. Articulation of our perspective, experience, and ideas is the human way of phenomenology.

Words are symbols to which man gives meaning as an outgrowth of his civilzation within his culture. Through words man attempts to communicatively describe his experienced states of being-in-his-world. In describing, of necessity, he relegates his uniquely known experiences to already known word symbols or categories. Thus, the conceptualized experience is limited, or less real than the lived unique experience. So, while words prevent the loss of the wisdom of lived experience, they are both a wonder of humanness and a limitation of humanness.

In describing human experiences there are efforts that can cut back this limitation. If we truly wish to convey meaning to others, really want to share what we have experienced in living, we will put forth the effort. To put forth such effort requires going beyond "I must publish to publish." It takes writing, structuring, rewriting, and restructuring often to a point where for a period one comes to hate materials he once held dear.

Through the years many of us come to use words as a means of passing a course, or we view words as a mode for self-explosion, expression, and self-understanding. In these ways they hold much purpose. The requirement that words convey unique experiences of being to others demands much more. This necessitates one selecting words that depict one's perspective, his unique human angular view; or depict for another, this particular man as he perceives and responds to his unique experience. Such a depiction has to be unknown to the other; each one's vantage point, given his history as an existent in this time and place, is singular. Then it requires finding words and putting them together in a way that best conveys the meaning the nursing event had to the nurse. An adequate dictionary and thesaurus can be useful.

The actual presentation of experience for an audience demands an ordering of data in a sequence that will be sensibly logical for them. We live experience in an order that flows from our being and history within a multiplicity of calls and responses. Presently human expression is limited to sequentiality. So again we see that the conceptualized experience is different from and lacks the reality of the uniquely lived event. Structuring a logical sequential presentation of data, deciding on those aspects that influenced meaning, and having it conform as closely as possible to the real is difficult.

Often, when it seems that one has done his very best, it is wise to have a trusted other react to conceptualizations. Another's questions can bring to the conceptualizer's awareness thought connections that moved him along and that he has failed to convey. Also, such a reader can indicate aspects of thought trips the writer took that add nothing to the issue at stake and weaken his message. Too, another's response can make apparent to a writer the need to clarify meaning. This clarification may merely entail a better choice of words or phrases, or it may suggest the use of a meaningful metaphor, analogy, or parable.

These last imaginative forms of expression we frequently use meaningfully, somethimes like a shorthand, with our intimates. A phrase, metaphor, or analogy conveys with an immediacy the quality or spirit of an event. For example, a nurse working in a psychiatric hospital unit speaking of a patient said, "He came down the hall looking like an accident about to happen." A page of technical description could not have given me as much feeling for what she and the patient were experiencing at that moment. In nurses' efforts to express objectively, scientifically, and eruditely such modes of expression are often deleted from our written professional works. It is as if we enforce the rules of medical record charting of precision, conciseness, and us of "weasel" words onto all our written works to the detriment of a theoretical and professional enduring body of nursing knowledge being actualized. It takes considerable pain and endeavor to find egress from such human programming. With it we have purified, equalized, wearied, and dehumanized supreme experiences of human existence. And, we have negated the meaning and importance of ourselves and nursing. How often have you heard, "I am *just* a nurse"?

Phenomenology requires rigorous investment into respectfully, appreciatively, and acceptingly making evident our lived worlds and their ramifications for the now, the past, and the anticipated future. Nursing literature of this caliber would call and inspire those who attended it to further nursing practice and responsibly share the meaning they attribute to their area of specialized dedication.

The raw data of our lived nursing worlds do not easily reveal their meanings or messages. Many see their worlds only superficially, and themselves as mere functions. How often a nurse is surprised, confounded, on hearing a relative or friend speak of a nursing event in their lives that may have occurred from 10 to 40 years previously. Frequently persons express appreciation for the meaning these events have had for them through the years. They remember the pleasure, anger, pain, fear, and/or joy they experienced.

It is not loose performance that allows raw data to convey its message to a nurse. New data are sucked easily and immediately into old, worn out, known theoretical frames and networks of words. Severe self-discipline enters into describing nursing experience with the vigor of how it was lived. Too easily the description is let fall to mediocre common forms. Proper grammar and plain English should suffice. This would carry the nursing message, as jargon borrowed from other disciplines in which the nurse always speaks as an alien, never will. Humanistic nursing practice theory in asking for description does not ask one to forget or deny known terms and knowledge. Rather it asks for a bracketing or holding of this knowledge to the side. The nursing experience should be given an opportunity to be seen in its pure form, rather than forcing it to conform to foreign presitigious terms borrowed from other areas of specialization, which beg the meaning of the nursing event. Prior to dispersion, of course, one should weigh one's expression in English against one's expression in one's known foreign jargon. Then one will be open to choose how one wants to express and share the meaning of her nursing world.

Phenomenology accepts categorization as a necessity of communicating. It holds, nevertheless, that this is secondary to intial aware experiencing. This study method acknowledges the unfathomable complexity of existing and knowing. It strives for as adequate conceptualization of the existential experience as possible. It honors the knowing person's continued capacity for surprise and wonderment. Phenomenology asks us to go beyond the common labels to the surprise of our own and other's unique existences-in-the-world. A nurse who had been struggling over many months with a family in their home, on the day she first experienced an "I-Thou" relationship with them said, "It was as if I had gone beyond the uncooperativeness and dirtiness of the situation." Immediacy in labeling offers us the complacency and security of a wrapped up problem. How could a nurse be held responsible for what happened to a "dirty," "uncooperative" family. The many commonly heard labels humans attribute inhumanely to others rarely relate to answers in situations or to the dreadful human suffering problems generate.

Phenomenology seeks attestation of the meaning of a situation to a participant. Positivism seeks general objective categories within the universal. Phenomenology prizes differences, variations, and struggles for their representation as parts of the whole. Rather than emphasize the majority as holding sway, it recognizes that the unique contribution can possibly be the weightiest in meaning.

THE PROCESS:
BECOMING A FREE RESPONSIBLE
RESEARCH NURSE

For a nurse to become a free responsible research nurse in the health arena she accepts her lived nursing world as beyond the controls valued in positivistic science. She appreciates her lived nursing world as saturated with knowledge to be extracted or wrung. Then she must examine, recognize, appreciate, and unfold her history, her angular view, and her human nurse potential. In prizing her view, as nurse, she will ask relevant nursing questions. To attain her potential as nurse she will discipline herself rigorously for authenticity with the self. With the self-acceptance that comes with self-authenticity she will know the importance of the difference she and the nursing profession make and can make in the community of man. Then out of her own human social need and for the survival of nursing she will describe to propel knowledge, nursing theory, and practice forward. In this process and in its effects she will become more human as she contributes to man's humanization.

6

THE LOGIC OF
A PHENOMENOLOGICAL METHODOLOGY

PERSPECTIVE: ANGULAR VIEW

In humanistic nursing practice theory we, Dr. Zderad and myself, propose that nursing practice when studied, like any other area studied, will only become available for human conceptualization if the study methods are appropriate to its nature. Therefore, the methodology presented in this chapter is relevant to humanistic nursing practice theory.

Embraced within this chapter is a methodology for studying nursing that evolved out of the process of my nursing practice. The logic of this method and of my process of nursing are one. It is not a method of another discipline superimposed on nursing. So this method did not force nursing or change nursing to have it mold or conform. As this method unfolded it arose from and in accord with nursing process. This methodology came into being only after years in which various attempts were made to get positivistic methodology to answer relevant nursing questions and to develop a professional scientific theory of nursing.

The method presented here was used initially to creatively conceptualize nursing constructs in 1967-68. The data for the development of the constructs "comfort" and "clinical" were gathered from my clinical nursing practice and while I was deeply engrossed in existential readings. The process or method used was not conceptualized until it was called for while writing my doctoral dissertation in 1968. It had then been used to study the clinical literary works of two psychiatric mental health nurses, Theresa G. Muller and Ruth Gilbert.[1] Its conceptualization at that time was rudimentary. Gradually it has been further conceptualized. "From a Philosophy of Nursing to a Method of

---

[1] Josephine G. Paterson, "Echo into Tomorrow: A Mental Health Psychiatric Philosophical Conceptualization of Nursing" D.N.Sc. dissertation, Boston University, 1969.

Nursology," an article published in *Nursing Research* in 1972, was my next attempt.[2] Graduate nursing students studied this article and repeated the process of the mehtodology in their studies of their clinical nursing data. Reflecting on this article and realizing how others had to study and struggle with it I became aware that still only the bare bones of my thinking were presented. Further elaboration of this methodology was called forth to share it with the *humanistic nursing practice theory* course participants. Since 1970 I have delved into phenomenologists' writings and at this time can say that this process of studying nursing is a phenomenologic method of nursology. Interesting to me is that the initiation of this method came when I first began to read the existentialist literature. Existentialism can be viewed as the fruits of phenomenological study. The process of this method has become clearer and clearer to me over time. Phenomenologically the process or method has grown out of the reality of the "thing itself" to be studied, in this case, clinical nursing practice.

This chapter then is the result of reflecting on these past efforts and is a conceptualization of this method as I understand it now.

The following quote is offered to support and validate the efforts put into conceptualizing this method. The philosopher of science Abraham Kaplan says of methodology:

> "The aim of methodology...is to invite speculation from science and practicality from philosophy...to help us understand in the broadest possible terms, not the products of scientific inquiry, but the process itself."[3]

The above quotation expresses the spirit in which this presentation is offered. Positivistic science aims at objectivity and its results are viewed as scientific facts. Nursing practice has been understood by many as an implementation of such theoretical facts. Considering my and other nurses' implementation of such facts it is apparent that in these endeavors nurses come to know much about human existence.

Philosophy is often viewed as man's contemplations, autobiographical revelations, and the values and belief systems that underlie man's actions, Can an explicit philosophy of nursing allow for more meaningful quality practice, be a resource for nurses, improve service, be available for reexemaination, correction, and the forwarding of knowledge? If nursing practice is viewed as the implementation of scientific facts and what they call forth in the nursing situation related to man's condition of existence, is a heuristic science of nursing developed from this situation, by nurses, an appropriate practical professional aim?

---

[2] Josephine G. Paterson "From a Philosophy of Clinical Nursing to a Method of Nursology," *Nursing Research* Vol. XX (March–April, 1971), pp. 143–146.

[3] Abraham Kaplan, *Conduct of Inquiry* (San Francisco: Chandler Publishing Co., 1964), p. 23.

This presentation is my answer, a committed "Yes."

The method offered here, a phenomenological method of nursology, aims at the reality of man, how he experiences his world, or it aims at a subjective-objective state. It aims at description of the professional clinical nursing situation which in reality is subjective-objective world that occurs between subjective-objective beings. The description focuses on this between and preserves the complex mobile flow of the river of nursing to make apparent that superficial precise portrayals are only an overlay of its river bed, course, and eventual destinations.

The relevance of phenomenological nursology ranges from the formulation of nursing constructs to the creation of theoretical propositions. It is applicable to one's own clinical data and to others' clinical data, here and now, or in historical study of the literature.

METHODOLOGICAL STARTING POINT

This method addresses itself to the question: How can a nurse, a subjective-objective human being know self and the other and compare and complementarily synthesize these known betweens?

Basic to this method is a belief system, a philosophy about the nature of man explicitly commented on by thinkers throughout human history.

Plato said:

> "I cannot be sure whether or not I see it as it really is; but we can be sure there is some such reality which it concerns us to see."[4]

Nurses are with other men in times of peak life experiences under the most intimate circumstances. We, too, can not be certain about what we come to know in our betweens. We can be sure that these realities of human experience are worthy of exploration. Our opportunities are unique, only we can describe man in the nursing situation.

In *Let Us Now Praise Famous Men,* James Agee voices a similar concern about the need to describe man-in-his-world and the adequacy of human description.[5] Aware of the wonders and complexities of man he considers not trying to describe worse than the inadequacy of description.

Thinkers have also acknowledged that we can come to know from others. A poem by Goethe expresses an attitude about this:

> "Somebody says: 'Of no school I am part,
> Never to living master lost my heart;
> Nor anymore can I be said
> To have learned anything from the dead.

---

[4] Plato, *The Republic,* trans. Francis MacDonald Cornford (New York: Oxford University Press, 1945), p. 45.

[5] James Agee, *Let Us Now Praise Famous Men* (New York: Ballantine Books, 1939), pp. 91–102.

That statement—subject to appeal—
Means: "I'm a self-made imbecile.' "[6]

In nursing what better master than the nursing situation in which we become through our relations with others. Each human person has something unique to teach us if we can but hear.

About our inadequacies of expression, many things are, are true, "all-at-once." The law of contradiction does not apply in-the-lived-experienced-world. We each view the world through our unique histories. Wisdom is many sided truth. Wisdom cannot be expressed "all-at-once." Truths can be stated only in sequence or metaphorically. If I were supercritical of my human limitations to express "all-at-once" wisdom, I would say nothing. Jung points up the dangers of this, he says:

"I must prevent my citical powers from destroying my creativeness. I know well enough that every word I utter carries with it something of myself—of my special and unique self with its particular history and its particular world."[7]

Each nurse's uniqueness dictates then a responsibility to share her particular knowing with fellow struggling human beings. Only through each describing can there be correction and complementary synthesis to movement beyond.

The nurse's world is an experiential place for becoming influenced by each participant's "here and now" inclusive or origin, history, and hopes, fears, and alternatives of the confronting future. Positivistic science focuses on selected particulars. Henri Bergson says:

". . .for us conscious beings, it is the units that matter, for we do not count extremities of intervals, we feel and live the intervals themselves."[8]

Each human participant in the nursing situation has a unique flow of consciousness which is intersubjectively influential.

So as human nurses we are limited in our ability to express the reality of our-lived worlds. Yet, also, this world depends on and demands that we, as human nurses, give it meaning, understand it in accordance with our

---

[6] Johann Wolfgang von Goethe, "On Originality." In *Great Writings of Goethe,* ed. Stephen Spender (New York: Mentor Press, 1958), p. 45.

[7] C.G. Jung, *Modern Man in Search of a Soul,* trans. W.S. Dell and Cary F. Baynes (New York: Harcourt, Brace and World, 1933), p. 118.

[8] Henri Bergson , "Time in the History of Western Philosophy," in *Philosophy in the Twentieth Century,* ed. William Barrett and Henry D. Aiken (New York: Random House, 1962), p. 252.

humanness. Will and Ariel Durant, historians, professionals who are forced to selectively present the world for other humans, say:

> "The historian will not mourn because he can see no meaning in human existence except that which man puts into it: let it be our pride that we ourselves may put meaning into our lives, and sometimes a significance that transcends death."[9]

Humans are the only beings conscious of themselves. Nurses are human beings. As such we are capable of looking at our existence, choosing our values, giving our world meaning and of constantly transcending ourselves, or becoming more. If we value and prize our human nursing world and our human potential for consciousness and expression, we will actuate our potential and conceptualize our human nurse-world. This suggests questions to me. What do I want nursing to be? How can I influence the meaning of the term, nursing? How committed am I? What investment am I willing to make? Will I risk exploring and saying what I see in my nursing world? Am I open to knowing? How can I actuate my uniqueness to allow the realistic potential of my nursing profession to become, become ever more? Am I contributing my "nursing here and now" to nursing's history through a lasting form of expression? Of what importance is what I think or say; do I make any difference? Hermann Hesse says of each man's uniqueness:

> "...every man is more than just himself; he also represents the unique, the very special and always significant and remarkable point at which the world's phenomena intersect, only once in this way and never again."[10]

Or, a nurse might say:

> "...every nurse is more than just herself, she also represents the unique, the very special and always significant and remarkable point at which the nursing world's phenomena intersect, only once in this way and never again."

To me, human freedom means recognizing our unique potential, responsibility, and limitations. Our singularity as a nurse among nurses, then, confronts us with a responsibility that belongs to one else. Martin Buber, philosophical anthropologist says:

> "As we become free...our responsibility must become personal and solitary."[11]

Our unlikeness to other nurses is a lonely, very person conditioned state. Only each nurse can be responsible for herself. The wonders of freedom are

---

[9] Will Durant and Ariel Durant, *Lessons of History* (New York: Simon and Schuster, 1968), p. 102.

[10] Hermann Hesse, *Demian,* trans. Michael Roloff and Michael Lebeck (New York: Harper & Row, 1965), p. 4.

[11] Martin Buber, *Between Man and Man,* trans. Ronald Gregor Smith (Boston: Beacon Press, 1955), p. 93.

paradoxically, "all-at-once," both a delight and a burden. In nursing it is important for us to understand freedom not as opposing or agreeing: freedom is choosing—choosing and saying "yes" to one's self.

Human endeavor between man and men in their-worlds, in this instance professional clinical nursing, if explored and described is viewed as contributing to man's human evolvement and to knowledge of the human condition and how man becomes.

Integrally all the above statements are the bases and biases of this human phenomenological method of nursology. In a phrase, I suppose what all these *starting point* statements say is : Nursing situations make available human existence events significantly worthy of description. Only human nurses can describe them. Humans' ability to describe reality adequately has its limits. We should describe since pridefully we humans are the only existing beings capable of giving meaning to, looking at, and expressing our consciousness. In the long run this effort could yield a nursing science.

PHASES OF PHENOMENOLOGIC NURSOLOGY

Phase I: Preparation of the Nurse Knower For Coming to Know

This method engages the investigator as a risk taker and as a "knowing place." Risk taking necessitates decision. Decision imposes confronting ambivalence in one's self. The ambivalence of wanting to be "all-at-once" responsible and dependent. Superimposing an already accepted and acceptable structure on data is safe feeling. Approaching the situation or data openly, letting the structure emerge from it, not deciding what to look for, being willing to be surprised, give feelings of excitment, fear, and uncertainty. There exists the possibility that our humanness may include the dilemma of our not being able to perceive the messages of our data, that we will not be able to merge with it and become more. The question arises, Are we knowing places that can relate to otherness and intuitively synthesize knowledge? This process of accepting the decision to approach the unknown openly is experienced as an internal struggle and we become consciously aware of our rigidity and satisfaction with the status quo. Conforming to the usual, in this case positivism, gives a security that is not easilty relinquished despite the advantages of actualizing our unique responsible freedom.

Russell's metaphorical phrase, "windows always open to the world," depicts the sought state of mind. His elaboration on this phrase gives the flavor of the process of preparing the mind. He says, "Through one's windows one sees not only the joy and beauty of the world, but also its pain and cruelty and ugliness, and the one is as well worth seeing as the other, and one must look into hell before one has any right to speak of heaven."[12] Pain, cruelty, ugliness, hell seem appropriate words to convey seeing our long-

---

[12] Bertrand Russell *The Autobiography of Bertrand Russell, 1914 – 1944* (Boston: Little, Brown and Co., 1968), p. 97.

cherished ideas and values, our security blankets, as only false gods. Nietzsche in speaking of confrontation of one's values said, "And now only cometh to him the great terror, the great outlook, the great sickness, the great nausea, the great seasickness."[13] So this human methodology seeks a condition of being in the investigator. The investigator must be aware of her own angular view and democratically open to giving the angular views apparent in the data, the called for representation.

The first phase of this method of research correlates well with the struggle experienced by me in clarifying my approach to patients in public health, medical-surgical, and psychiatric mental health situations. In these situations, one truly has to struggle with democratically keeping one's windows open to the world. And this is a continual process. Having experienced this struggle in clincal nursing made this approach to research valid and meaningful to me.

Preparing the mind for knowing in clinical or research endeavors may be accomplished by several means. One means is by immersing one's self in dramatic and literary works and contemplating, reflecting on, and discussing them as they relate to the knower's already known, in this case, nursing practice. In clinical or research nursing the selection of literary works to stimulate the opening of one's human view is based on their presentation, depictions, and descriptions of man's nature. In literature authors share their thoughts as men and present possible ways men may view and relate to their worlds.

Phase II: Nurse Knowing of the Other Intuitively

Bergson conceives of man knowing through a dilatation of his imagination getting inside of, into *le durée,* into the rhythm and mobility of the other. Living the rhythm of the other he believes results in an absolute, intuitive, inexpressible, unique knowledge of the other. He says:

"...an absolute can only be given in an intuition, while all the rest has to go with analysis."

"...from intuition one can pass on to analysis, but not from analysis to intuition."

"...fixed concepts can be extracted by our thought from the mobile reality; but there is not means whatever of reconsituting with the fixity of concepts the mobility of the real."[14]

The known, clinical nursing practice, gave meaning to the above for me. Over the years in nursing conferences I had been told my grasp of nursing situations was intuitive. Most times this was offered rather disparagingly although the nursing outcomes were most times successful. Along with having

---

[13] Frederick Nietzsche "Thus Spake Zarathustra," trans. Thomas Common, in *The Philosophy of Nietzsche* (New York: Random House, 1927), p. 239.

[14] Henri Bergson, "An Introduction to Metaphysics," In *Philosophy in the Twentieth Century,* ed. William Barrett and Henry D. Aiken (New York: Random House, 1962), pp. 303–331.

the attribute of intuition assigned to me persons often asked, "Why are you so fascinated with other persons' situations?" Together these relate to Dewey's view of intuition. He views intuition as a mulling over of conditions and a mental synthesis that results in true judgments since the controlling standards are intelligent selection, estimation, and problem solution.[15] In nursing practice research knowing the other and how he experiences and views his world is viewed as the problem.

Knowing intuitively, as described by Bergson, is comparable to Buber's considerations of man's necessary mode of becoming through "I-Thou" relation. The criteria Buber describes as characteristic for "I-Thou" relation are subscribed to in my approach to nursing practice and in this human or phenomenological nursology approach.[16] Buber held as prerequisite for intuitive type knowing of the other, or imagining the real of his potential for being, a knower, and "I," capable of distance from the other, able to see the other as a unique other, one who turns to the other, makes his being present to the other, and allows the other presence. The knowing, "I," in this case the nurse, responds to the other's uniqueness, does not superimpose, maintains a capacity for surprise and question, and is with the other, as opposed to "seeming to be." This kind of relating cannot be superimposed on a nurse clinician or researcher. It must be personally responsibly chosen and invested in.

The approach then of the second phase of this method and of the transactional phase of nursing when nurses are in the arena with others is the same. This method proposes that to study nursing from outside the arena for purposes of objectivity bursts assunder the very nature of nursing practice. The studier is a part of that which is being studied. Observations interpreted from outside the situation could be classified only as projections.

Phase III: Nurse Knowing the Other Scientifically

Bergson believes man knows incompletely through standing outside the thing to be known, metaphorically walking around it, and observing it. This analytical process, this viewing of a thing's many aspects, he conceives as the habitual function of positive science. This is the third phase of this phenomenological nursology method. Bergson says:

"...analysis multiplies endlessly the points of view...to complete the ever incomplete representation."

"All analysis is thus a translation, a development into symbols, a representation taken from successive points of view."

"Analysis...is the operation which reduces the object to elements already known, that is, common to that object and to others."[17]

---

[15] John Dewey, *How We Think* (Boston: D.C. Heath & Co., Publishers, 1910), p. 105.
[16] Martin Buber, "Distance and Relation," trans. Ronald Gregor Smith, in *The Knowledge of Man,* ed. Maurice Friedman. (New York: Harper & Row, Publishers, 1965), pp. 60–82.
[17] Bergson, *"An Introduction to Metaphysics,"* pp. 303–331.

So phenomenological nursology proposes that after the studier has experienced the other intuitively and absolutely, tne experience be conceptualized and expressed in accordance with the nurse's human potential. Humanly we can express only sequentially while our actual experienced lived worlds flow in an "all-at-once" fashion. Our words are known symbols and categories used to convey the experience and thus deny the uniqueness of each realized experience.

Buber's description of man's "I-It" way of relating to the world is in agreement with Bergson. He conveys the necessity of this kind of relating by man to his world; and despite its lacks proposes that man prize his analytical ability. Like Bergson, Buber views knowing as a movement from intuition to analysis, and not the other way around. Buber sees knowledge expressed or science created through the knowing "I" transcending itself, recollecting, reflecting on, and experiencing its past "I-Thou" relation as an "It." This is man being conscious of, looking at, himself and that which he has taken in, merged with, made part of himself. This is the time when he mulls over, analyzes, sorts out, compares, contrasts, relates, interprets, gives a name to, and categorizes.

The third phase of this methodology is the same as that phase of clinical nursing practice in which the nurse, removed from the nursing arena, replays and reflects on this area and transcribes her angular view of it. In this reflective state the nurse analyzes, considers relationships between components, synthesizes themes or patterns, and then conceptualizes or symbolically interprets a sequential view of this past lived reality. The challenge of communicating a lived nursing reality demands authenticity with the self and rigorous effort in the selection of words, phrases, and precise grammar.

Phase IV:
Nurse Complementarily Synthesizing Known Others

In this phase of the methodology the nurse researcher, the knower, compares and synthesizes multiple known realities. Buber says of comparison:

> "The act of contrasting, carried out properly and adequately, leads to the grasp of the principle."[18]

In this comparison and synthesis the "I" of the researcher assumes the position of the knowing place. The knower, like an interpreter, allows dialogue between the multiple known realities. These realities are unknowable to each other directly. The knower interprets, sorts, and classifies.

In the human knowing place discovered differences in similar realities do not compete, one does not negate the other. Each can be true, present, "all-at-once." Differences can make visible the greater realities of each. Desan, the philosopher, says of this kind of synthesis:

---

[18] Martin Buber, *I and Thou,* 2nd ed., trans. Ronald Gregor Smith, (New York: Charles Scribner's Sons, 1958). pp. 3–34.

"...a synthetic view where two or more positions are seen to illuminate and to transfigure one another through their mutual presence."[19]

The knower alert to an aspect present in a single reality can question the other reality on this aspect. This aspect may be present in both, more blatant in one than in another. Its forms may be different or modified in each. It may be totally absent in one. Differences found may arouse or bring to consciousness other questions to ask of the data. This oscilating, dialectical process continues throughout reflection on the multiple realities. This indirect dialogue is recorded by the investigator as the complementary synthesis.

This synthesis is more than additive because it allows mutual representation and the illumination of one reality by another.

The fourth phase of this research methodology is like that phase of clinical nursing in which a nurse compares and synthesizes the similarities and differences of like nursing situations and arrives at an expanded view.

Phase V: Succession Within the Nurse From the Many to the Paradoxical One

This phase of phenomenological nursology is highly probable if not absolutely necessary. Desan says:

"Truth emerges in and through the relational operation. For the way of paradox is the way of truth."[20]

The investigator may struggle with the multiplicity of views now consciously part of and within herself. Again Desan:

"...this unrest "is" the mind of man, reaching its center. ...From this center the splendor of multiplicity is visible."[21]

The researcher, mulling over and considering the relationships between the multiple views, insightfully corrects and expands her own angular view. This is not a right-wrong type of correction. Such correction would amount only to an ongoing eternal recurrence of a frustrating nature. Rather this correction takes the form of ever more inclusiveness. Struggling with the communion of the different ideas the knower takes an intuitive leap, through and yet beyond these ideas, into a greater understanding. She then may come up with a conception or abstraction that is inclusive of and beyond the multiplicities and contradictions.

This inclusive conception or abstraction is an expression of the investigator in her here and now, with the old truths and the novel truths, none obliterated.

---

[19] W.D. Desan, *Planetary Man* (New York: The Macmillan Company, 1972), p. 77.
[20] *Ibid.*
[21] *Ibid.* p. 80.

The fifth phase of this phenomenological nursology method can be equated to that phase of clinical professional nursing in which the nurse propels nursing knowledge forward. In this phase a nurse struggling with the mutual communion of multiple nursing situations arrives at a conception that is meaningful to the many or to all. From the specific concrete ideas of the many situations she moves through dilemma to resolution which is nursing expressed abstractly in units or as a whole, as one.

Experiential knowledge of nursing, years in which I came to know self and the other while implementing scientific facts, allowed me as a knower to recognize the relevance of this philosophical nursology method. This method does not aim at conventionality. Rather it strives to meaningfully augment and share conceptualized nurse–world realities.

7

A PHENOMENOLOGICAL APPROACH TO HUMANISTIC NURSING THEORY

Humanistic nursing is dialogical in the theoretical as well as the practical realm. Just as the meaning of humanistic nursing is found in the existential intersubjective act, that is, in the dialogue as it is lived out by nurse and patient in the real world, so the theory of humanistic nursing is formed in the dialogical interplay of articulated experiences shared by searching, abstracting, conceptualizing nurses.

The theory of humanistic nursing originates from and is continually revitalized and refined by actual nursing experience. But each nurse, as a unique human being, necessarily experiences the nursing dialogue and her nursing world in a unique way. So the development of humanistic nursing theory rests on the sharing of individual unique angular views. And the theory as a totality will become richer, more consonant with reality, as it represents more and more nurses' views.

So often nurses, even nurses who know that their clinical expertise grew out of their practice, hesitate to share their nursing experiences. They are apt to say deprecatingly, "Oh, that's *only* my *personal* experience." Yet that is precisely where the value lies, in the uniqueness of human experience. Since each nurse's description of her nursing experience is a glimpse of a real nursing world, the views cannot justifiably be judged as right or wrong; they simply are. Once the various views are expressed, they can be compared and contrasted, not for the purpose of accepting some and rejecting others but rather in the interest of clarifying each in relation to the other. Such a dialogue of experientially based conceptualizations can result in a complementary synthesis. The process calls for not only a true appreciation of personal experience by each nurse but also commitment to a collaborative effort of open sharing by a genuine community of nurses.

This view, that the development of humanistic nursing practice theory is a dialogical process, has led to our valuing (in fact, insisting on) the description of nursing phenomena. We see phenomenological description as a basic and essential step in theory building. Indeed, considering the "state-of-the-art" of nursing theory development, it is the most crucial and immediate need.

Looking back at the historical evolvement of our humanistic nursing approach, it is obvious that we had been using and developing a phenomenological approach for a number of years before we graced our efforts with the impressive label, "Phenomenological Psychiatric Mental Health Nursing," in a course offered to a group of nurses at Northport Veterans Administration Hospital in April 1972. Although we were aware much earlier that our interests and work were flowing in the general stream of phenomenology, we usually refrained from using the label because it did little to clarify our position.[1] The term has grown less precise with the extension of its use in different disciplines and with variations in methodology.

When we began applying the term "phenomenological" to our work, we learned that to many persons it sounds strange, unpronounceable, foreign; to some forbidding; to others enticing. We later coined the title "humanistic nursing" as being more suitable for it encompasses our general existential bent. However, this change in title does not imply any abandonment of our phenomenological approach. The description of nursing phenomena is as highly prized now as ever. In humanistic nursing, phenomenological and existential currents interrelate. Having an existential view of nursing as a living dialogue influences which phenomena one becomes aware of, experiences, values, studies, and describes. Reciprocally, as one discovers and struggles to describe and develop meaningful ways of describing nursing phenomena, the lived nursing dialogue itself will be continually perfected.

It is more precise to speak of phenomenological methods (in the plural) rather than phenomenological method (in the singular), for, since Edmund Husserl's original work, the the approach has been used by different desciplines. With its spread there has developed a corresponding variation in methodology. This, in a sense, is the beauty of phenomenology: it thrives on variety of perspective; it allows, perhaps requires, individual creativeness; it is always open. In this spirit, ideas are offered here with the hope of stimulating imaginative, critical response, and further development of methodology.

This chapter considers some of the more concrete deatils of phenomenological methodology as they relate to humanistic nursing. The general approach and procedures discussed below have been used, individually

---

[1] Loretta T. Zderad, "A Concept of Empathy" (Ph.D. dissertation, Georgetown University, 1968). Josephine G. Paterson, "Echo into Tomorrow: A Mental Health Psychiatric Philosophical Conceptualization of Nursing" (D.N.Sc. dissertation, Boston University, 1969). Loretta T. Zderad, "Empathy—From Cliche to Construct," *Proceedings of the Third Nursing Theory Conference* (University of Kansas Medical Center Department of Nursing Education, 1970), pp. 46–75. Josephine G. Paterson, "From a Philosophy of Clinical Nursing to a Method of Nursology," *Nursing Research,* Vol. XX (March–April, 1972), pp. 143–146. Josephine G. Paterson and Loretta T. Zderad, "All Together Through Complementary Synthesis," *Image,* Vol. IV, No.3 (1970–71), pp. 13–16.

and collaboratively, by Dr. Josephine Paterson and myself with individual and groups of nurses to explore and describe their nursing experiences. They have helped nurses in various levels and types of nursing service to take a fresh look at their practice and make desirable changes. We have lived through the process with graduate students in nursing, and it has led both the students and us to new conceptualizations and reconceptualizations of nursing phenomena. We have found this to be a fruitful research method when applied to clinical nursing phenomena personally experienced and/or reported in the literature. And we are currently exploring its potentials with interested nurses at Northport Veterans Administration Hospital.

A PHENOMENOLOGICAL APPROACH

The method may be characterized generally as descriptive but it is not a simple cataloguing of qualities or counting of elements. Basically, it involves an openness to nursing phenomena, a spirit of receptivity, readiness for surprise, the courage to experience the unknown. Equally important is awareness of one's own perspective and of personal biases. The methodological process is subjective–objective and intuitive–analytic. Besides subjective knowing or personal experiencing of the phenomenon, rigorous analysis also is required. This being-with (subjective, intuitive knowing and experiencing) and looking at (objective analyzing) the phenomenon all at once sparks a creative synthesis, a conceptualization from which emanates insightful description.

More specifically, the method entails *an intuitive grasp of the phenomenon, analytic examination of its occurrences, synthesis, and description.* In actuality, as the method is carried out, one does not necessarily recognize or focus on these processes as distinct phases or steps. In the flow of the experience, at times, some seem to occur simultaneously or in oscillation. Bearing this in mind, the processes will be considered in more detail.

Intuitive Grasp of the Phenomenon

Phenomenology is grounded in experience. It values the raw data of immediate experience. ("To the things themselves," was the slogan that inspired and guided Husserl and his followers.) So this approach requires, in the first place, attitudes of openness and awareness. It involves learning to become conscious of spontaneous perceptions, or in other words, getting in touch with one's sensations and feelings. It means capturing prereflective experience, that is, becoming aware of one's immediate impression or response to reality before labeling, categorizing, or judging it.

In this kind of a state of readiness to receive what appears, a phenomenon may be grasped intuitively. It is as if a particular bit of reality, a happening, flashes *impressively* into one's awareness. The intensity of the experience and the absorption of one's attention in the phenomenon vary over a wide range. There may be only a fleeting recognition of a phenomenon accompanied by a half-formulated thought or judgment, such as, "hmm, that's interesting," with immediate dismissal from or replacement of it by something else in one's consciousness. The impression may, of course, be stored in memory and pop out again at a later time. Or the phenomenon may strike on one's consciousness more forcefully causing further pondering and wonder. Or the impression of the phenomenon may be so startling that it fills one's consciousness to the point of pushing all else out; a person is momentarily "stopped in his tracks."

In the intuitive grasp, regardless of its intensity or duration, the phenomenon appears clear and distinct. The intuitive grasp is an insight into reality that bears the certainty of immediate experience. No discursive process intervenes; one simply knows the phenomenon as it is experienced. Furthermore, the intuitive grasp provides a kind of definite and whole understanding, a gestalt, that allows recognition of the phenomenon in other situations. So when the person is faced with another event he can say, "Yes, that is the phenomenon under consideration, " or "No, that is not it."

In order to be open to the data of experience in using a phenomenological approach, one strives to eliminate "the *a priori*" (that which exists in his mind prior to and independent of the experience). This is done by attempting to "bracket" (hold in abeyance) theoretical presuppositions, interpretations, labels, categories, judgments, and so forth. Granted, a person cannot be completely perspectiveless. Man is an individual; he is a unique here and now person. So naturally, *necessarily,* he has an "angular" view for he experiences reality from the angle of his own particular "here" and his own particular "now." Or, stated differently, as a knowing, experiencing subject, each man must have *some* perspective of the phenomenon being experienced. However, by recognizing and considering the particular perspective from which he is experiencing it, a person may become more open to the thing itself.

Furthermore, this kind of openness to one's own perspective can be developed through deliberate practice. Several approaches may be used. To begin with, a person can develop the habit of recognizing and exposing his own biases. This could involve something as basic as stating the actual physical situation or circumstance in which the phenomenon was experienced. For example: the phenomenon could be something seen from above or below, at a distance or nearby; something heard in a quiet room or above the din of background noise; a patient's behavior in a large group or in a small group, with his family, with on particular nurse, with his doctor; a patient's response while being fed, bathed, monitored.

Beyond this unavoidable bias of the angle of perception, the nurse's experience of her lived world may be dulled by habituation. It is necessary to break through the tunnel vision of routine. For instance, a nurse new to a situation may notice a patient's response to her and remark about it to another nurse. The second nurse, to whom the patient's behavior is familiar, may respond, "Oh, he's done that for years." Often this is the end of the dialogue;it should be the beginning, for the duration of a phenomenon is not equal to its description or meaning, but rather, is an indication of its significance.

The mystery of the commonplace is hidden by veils of the obvious. To recognize one's biases means to put one's beliefs, one's cherished notions, out on the table. A helpful aid in reflecting on and articulating an experience is the question, "What am I taking for granted?" Commonly used terms, such as, "psychiatric patient," "orthopedic patient," "oncology unit," "un-cooperative," "emotional," "chronic," "terminal," "hopeless," "outpa-tient," "ambulatory," "visitors," "family," "doctor," "nurse," "ad-ministration," "front office" have an aura of connotations that may corres-pond to or differ greatly from the actual immediate experience. It may be a case where believing is seeing. The habit of premature labeling may close a person to the full savoring of experience.

Another means of increasing openness to one's own perspective is to con-sciously note whether the phenomenon is being experienced actively or passively. For example, the phenomenon may be the motion of changing a patient's position in bed. Both experience the motion, but it is a different ex-perience for the nurse who actively moves the patient and for the patient who is moved passively. Or again, many studies of the phenomenon of empathy have been reported in the literature. Almost exclusively, these are descriptions of empathizing with someone; only rarely are they concerned with the ex-perience of being empathized with. Yet obviously, the active and passive ex-periences of the phenomenon of empathy are different. The same holds true for touching and being touched, bathing and being bathed, feeding and being fed, supporting and being supported, reassuring and being reassured, and many other phenomena in nursing.

Similarly, awareness of one's perspective may be increased by consciously realizing whether the phenomenon is being viewed objectively or subjectively. Consider for example, phenomena such as pain, anxiety, sleep, restlessness, boredom. Seeing evidence of pain in another person is not the same as feeling pain within myself. Recognizing objective signs of anxiety in another person differs from the subjective experience of feeling anxious myself. Sleeping and observing someone sleeping are two different experiences. The same hold true for restlessness, boredom, and so forth.

In view of nursing's dialogical character it may be assumed that many phenomena of major concern would be intersubjective or transactional. It is important then for nurses, attempting to develop openness to their own perpectives, to consider whether the phenomenon involves two subjects and their between. Does the action go both ways? Are both persons calling and responding to each other simultaneously? Take the phenomenon of "timing" for example. The nurse's verbal response to a patient depends not only on her perception of her own here-and-now and his perception of his here-and-now but rather it aslo involves their perceptions of their shared here-and-now situa-tion. The nursing world is filled with intersubjective phenomena such as, eye contact, touch, silence. To describe these fully the nurse must be open to her perspective, the patient's perspective, and their between.

Analysis, Synthesis, and Description

After a nursing phenomenon is grasped intuitively, it is desirable to find as many instances of it as possible for the sake of description. Keeping the phenomenon in mind and reflecting on it from time to time, the nurse becomes more alert to its occurrence in her lived world. The phenomenon may be experienced directly. In which case, it is described and reflected on and descriptions, reflections, and questions are recorded. When she observes the phenomenon in others, the nurse may ask them to describe it and verify her own observations. Some nurses have involved other staff members in discovering and describing instances of the phenomenon being studied. Similarly, one becomes more open to descriptions of it in the literature—any literature—or in any form of human expression, for example, poetry, drama, art, science. As many descriptions of the phenomenon are gathered from as many angles a possible, these are the data to be analytically examined, synthesized, and described.

The three processes of analysis, synthesis, and description are so interrelated and so intertwined in reality that it is simpler to discuss techniques in relation to all three. Some techniques are equally useful in the analytic examination and the description of phenomena. In a sense, a person does both at once. And often, it is during this process of shifting back and forth, analyzing and describing an experience that synthesis occurs. A person gets a sudden insight, "everything falls into place," "it clicks." One gets a gestalt, a whole, not necessarily a whole in the sense of complete and entire, but a whole frame, form, or structure that allows for further developing and filling in of details.

There are many ways of going about the analysis and description. The following are some that have been found useful in the expliction of nursing phenomena.

Comparing and contrasting instances of the phenomenon lead to the discovery of similarities and differences. For instance, in studying patients' crying it was found that their crying was with or without tears; loud or silent; expressing pain, anger, fear, sorrow. Or again, silence may be defined simply as absence of sound. But silence as experienced in the real nursing world has other chracteristics. It may convy anger, fear, peacefulness, and so forth. It is these nuances or qualities of silence that are significant cues for the nursing dialogue. They could be brought to light by comparing and contrasting descriptions of silence.

Various instances of the phenomenon being studied may be examined to discover common elements. Characteristics or elements seen in one instance are sought in the others. For example, when descriptions of interpersonal empathy were scrutinized, it became evident that in all cases there were physiological, psychological, and social components. Examining experiences of reassurance revealed they had elements such as empathy, sympathy, reality orientation, feelings of hope and comfort.

One may determine which elements are essential to the phenomenon by imaginative variation, that is, by trying to imagine the phenomenon without a particular element. For instance, reassurance without empathy or sympathy would be false reassurance or, in other words, would not reassure.

The elements of the phenomenon can be studied to determine how they are interrelated. One may ask, is there a priority in time? Does one element develop from another? Consider the phenomenon of reassurance; does empathy precede sympathy? Or, to take another example, in the empathic experience, an openness to the other and an imaginative projection into his place lead to the vicarious experiencing of his situation.

For further clarification of its distinctive qualities the phenomenon may be related to and distinguished from other similar phenomena. For example, empathy is similar to and also different from identification, projection, compassion, sympathy, love, and encounter.

By considering what it has in common with other phenomena, the phenomenon being described may be classified as being subsumed in a broader category. Thus, empahty is a human response, a coalescent movement, a form of relating.

The phenomenon may be described by selecting its central or decisive characteristics and abstracting its accidentals. For instance, interpersonal empathy always involves movement into another's perspective and as a form of movement it has directions, dimensions, and degrees. It can occur between persons of difference age, education, experience, sex; these latter characteristics are accidental.

Some descriptions make use of negation. A phenomenon cannot be described completely by negation but it may be clarified to some extent by saying what it is not. For instance, empathy is not sympathy; it is not projection; it is not identification.

Analogy may be used to promote analytic examination and description. This involves a comparison based on partial similarity between like features of two things. For example, the movement of empathy is like the currents in the sea; the heart is like a pump. The advantage of using analogy is that the comparison raises questions about the nature of the phenomenon under consideration. However, since the similarity between the analogues is always partial, one must guard against overextending the comparison to unwarranted conclusions. The description must always be consonant with the phenomenon as it occurs in reality.

The use of a metaphor also may enhance description and analysis. A metaphor suggests comparison of the phenomenon with another by the nonliteral application of a word. For example, "the between is a secret place." The use of metaphor may be criticized in regard to its lack of precision. On the other hand, there are some (for example, Marcel, Buber) who hold that the intersubjective realm can be described only metaphorically because it is beyond the level of objectivity. And to attempt to describe intersubjective phenomena in precise terms related to the physical world would tend to distort rather than clarify. Many of the nursing phenomena requiring description occur within the intersubjective realm. Metaphors could cast some light on these.

CONCLUSION

As a theory of practice, humanistic nursing is derived from individual nurses' actual experiences in their uniquely perceived but commonly shared nursing world. Its development, therefore, depends on the articulation of their angular views and also on the truly collaborative effort of a genuine community of nurses struggling together to describe humanistic nursing practice.

Since the description of nursing phenomena is recognized as a basic and essential step in theory development, this chapter presented an approach and detailed some techniques used by nurses to describe phenomena. It is hoped that these would be viewed critically and creatively; that they would be used, varied, combined adapted, and lead to new methods suited to the description of nursing phenomena. And if they are developed, it is hoped that they will be shared for the growth of humanistic nursing depends not only on using and sharing what we learn but also on describing how we come to know. Then humanistic nursing theory will grow in dialogue.

8

HUMANISTIC NURSING AND ART

The term "humanistic nursing" often is interpreted as implying humane-ness. Logically, humane caring must be one aspect (a major aspect) or a natural expression of humanistic nursing practice theory. But the term means more. According to the position being taken here, nursing may be described appropriately as humanistic since at its very base it is an inter-human event. As an intersubjective transaction, its meaning is found in the human situation in which it occurs. As an existential act, it involves all the participants' capacities and aims at the development of human potential, that is, at well-being and more-being. Our approach qualifies, then, as a form of humanism, according to the dictionary definition, being "a system or mode of thought or action in which human interests, values, and dignity are taken to be of primary importance."

In another sense of the word, our theoretical stance is humanistic by virtue of its regard for the humanities and arts. Philosophy, literature, poetry, drama, and othe forms of art are valued as resources for enriching our knowledge of man and the human situation. They also are seen as suitable means for expressing or describing the lived realities of the nurse's world.

Contemporary nursing, being a true child of its time, reflects American society's high regard for "Science." Values of science are easily discernible in nursing and affect the character of its research, education, and practice. Consider, for instance, how the nursing dialogue is influenced by the prizing of objectivity, precision of language, operational definitions, scientific jargon, development of constructs and theories, methodology of scientific inquiry, emphasis on quantification and measurement.

There is much more written in our current literature about nursing as a science than about nursing as an art. Although slighted, the humanities have not been rejected. In fact, some nurses and educators are urging that the role

85

of the humanities and arts be recognized in nursing and that they be used more effectively in undergraduate and graduate nursing education.[1]

Turning to my own personal experience, I recall that one of the first definitions I had to learn in my basic nursing program began with the statement, "Nursing is an art and science. . ." (It is interesting that now, years later, this is all I can recall of the definition!) At that time, I accepted the statement at face value. I did not question it. Perhaps I had not thought enough about art and science and certainly I did not know enough about nursing to question the description. Yet over the years many experiences and insights have turned into questions that challenge this adopted cherished notion.

In the beginning I merely accepted the view that nursing is an art in the sense of being a skillful or aesthetic application of scientific principles. After all, we had a course in nursing arts (later called fundamentals of nursing). This had to do with bathing, feeding, making beds, and hundreds of other nursing procedures that were presented as "nursing arts," the doing of nursing. At the time I also had courses in the humanities and liberal arts. These courses were not related directly to nursing by either the teachers or myself, as I recall. I did not ask: In what way is nursing an art? What kind of art is nursing? Or, how does the art of nursing differ from other arts?

The notion (perhaps "conviction" would be more accurate) that nursing is an art in some sense other than an artful application of scientific principles has been with me for a long time. I do not know its origin nor even the form in which the view first appealed to me. I do recall having difficulty on several occasions in trying to express let alone explain, my idea. At these times, what I experienced subjectively as an intuitive flash of insight would end up objectified in an amorphous blob of words. Yet the theme returns over and over in a variety of questions and issues that demand response if not resolution. This chapter offers some further reflections on the relatedness of humanistic nursing and art.

USE OF ARTS

One of the most obvious ways in which nursing and art are related is in nursing's use of the arts. This may be seen in nursing education as well as in nursing practice.

---

[1] New England Council on Higher Education for Nursing, *Humanities and the Arts as Bases for Nursing:* Implications for Newer Dimensions in Generic Nursing Education, Proceedings of the Fifth Inter-University Work Conference (Lennox, Mass: New England Council on Higher Education for Nursing, June, 1968). "Humanities, Humaneness, Humanitarianism," Editorial in *Nursing Outlook*, Vol. 18, No. 9 (September, 1970), p. 21. Charles E. Berry and E.J. Drummond, "The Place of the Humanities in Nursing Education," *Nursing Outlook,* Vol. 18, No. 9 (September, 1970), pp. 30-31. Marion E. Kalkman, "The Role of the Humanities in Graduate Programs in Nursing," in *Doctoral Preparation for Nurses,* ed. Esther A. Garrison (San Francisco: University of California, 1973), pp. 138-155.

Liberalization

Usually, when arts and humanities are included in nursing education programs, it is for their humanizing effects. Traditionally they have been recognized as having a civilizing influence. So in nursing they are seen as supporting the elements of humaneness and humanitarianism. Furthermore, they are a necessary antidote for the depersonalization that accompanies scientific technology and mechanization.

The arts are valued also for their liberalizing effect. They stimulate imaginative creativity. They broaden a person's perspective of the human situation, of man in his world. For instance, depictions of suffering man or of other aspects of the human condition that are found in poetry, drama, or literature are far more descriptive and much closer to reality than those given in typical textbooks.

Current nursing practice reflects the educational peparation of nurses that is weighted heavily with sceintific courses and the methodology of positivistic science. Arts and humanities are a necessary complement. Science aims at universals and the discovery of general laws; art reveals the uniqueness of the individual. While science strives for quanitification, art is more concerned with quality. Strict conformance to methodology and replicability are prized in scientific studies, whereas freedom and uniqueness of style reign in art. Science, forever updating itself, opens the nurse's eyes to constant change and innovation; the classics promote a sense of the unchanging and lasting in man's world. Science may provide the nurse with knowledge on which to base her decision, but it remains for the arts and humanities to direct the nurse toward examination of values underlying her practice. Thus, humanistic nursing has both scientific and artistic dimensions.

Expression

Humanistic nursing and art are interrelated in another way. Some nurses who are also artists use their respective arts to express their nursing experience. Poetry is a good example.

In an article, "Nurses as Poets," Trautman notes that since the 1940s progressively greater numbers of poems about nursing have been published and since the 1960s the quality of these poems has improved considerably.[2] She believes that nurses' ability to express their feelings about nursing in poetry cannot be attributed entirely to a change in times. Rather, it is a reflection of change in nursing practice. For one thing, contemporary nursing requires a great deal of abstract thinking. It calls for an understanding involving mental and emotional investment, and imaginative feeling *with* the patient. The

---

[2] Mary Jane Trautman, "Nurses as Poets," *American Journal of Nursing,* Vol. 71, No. 4 (April, 1971), p.727.

nurse-poet puts aside technical terms, looks at her patient in a fresh and creative way and shares her view in a poem.

A second reason offered by Trautman is the increased emphasis in nursing education on communication and verbal skills. A nurse with a talent for writing may be moved by a particular experience to share it. Thus, "the sensitive nurse-writer may use poetic expression to work through a problem, to muse about a detail, or to record a profound experience."[3]

Finally, she states that some nurses write poetry about aspects of their work that defy scientific analysis and cannot be easily contained in technical papers. In this, then, nurses' poetry goes beyond the personal satisfaction accompanying expression; it preserves a unique angular view of nursing's lived world and adds to our store of clinical wisdom. As Trautman concludes:

"Poetry has trailed the profession for many years, probably because nurses were not encouraged in creative writing of any kind. Today, however, I think that poetry leads the profession because most of it never loses sight of human needs—both nurses' and patients'. Our poets lend a clear and vital voice to our profession. They cite their experiences, emotions, beliefs, and awareness in lieu of a science-oriented bibliography. They appeal to our common sense but, more importantly to our hearts. They tell us to observe honestly and to feel. Above all, our poets tell us to believe in our observations and to trust in our feelings—for patients, for ourselves."[4]

Some elements or aspects of nursing lend themselves to scientific exploration and discovery while others, equally important and likewise deserving expression, reveal themselves only through the artist's vision. So what has been said of poetry, therefore, may hold true in other arts. Each art has its own form of dialogue with reality. The painter, for example, feels with his eyes; he feels lines, points, planes, texture, and color.[5] What could the nurse-painter share? Or as Garner, a nurse-musician, suggests, nursing could be conceptualized along the schema of tones, texture, rhythm, meter, intensity, temperament.[6]

What nursing content would accrue if the various nurse-artists used their forms of knowledge, skill, and vision to explore nursing as the various nurse-scientists do? What can our poets, painters, musicians and dancers see, hear, feel in the nursing dialogue?

Therapeutics

There is a third way in which humanistic nursing and art are related. For many years, the arts have been used in nursing for their therapeutic effects, especially with psychiatric, geriatric, and pediatric patients. The nurse and a patient or a group of patients participate in an artistic experience together. These may be passive activities,such as, attending a concert or play or visiting

---

[3] *Ibid.,* p. 728.
[4] Ibid.
[5] Chaim Potok, *My Name Is Asher Lev* (Greenwich, Conn.: Fawcett Publications, 1972), p. 105.
[6] Grayce C. Scott Garner, "Qualitative and Quantitative Analyses of Schizophrenic Verbal and Non-Verbal Acts Related to Selected Kinds of Music," *Humanities and the Arts,* p. 49.

an art exhibit; or they may be active ones in which nurse and patients are involved in artistic expression or creation.

Music, poetry, painting, drama, and dance have been used effectively in various nursing situations. For instance, Christoffers, a nurse and dancer, emphasizes the importance of body language as communication and supports her view with clinical evidence. She urges nurses to become "physically literate—to develop an understanding and appreciation of the part played by body language in human relationships."[7] Or again, according to Garner, "Music, when carefully planned, can be used as a source of culture, nurturance, communication, socialization, and therapeusis."[8]

A major therapeutic value of art lies in the fact that it confronts one with reality. "Art is a lie which makes us realize the truth."[9] In his novel, *The Conspiracy,* Hersey has Lucan, a poet, write to Seneca:

> "To me the ideal of a work of art is that each man should be able, in contemplating it, to see himself as he really is. Thus art and reality meet. This is the great healing strength of art, this is the power of art,...Art's power which nothing can challenge, is the blinding light of recognition."[10]

By using various art forms the nurse helps the patient experience, become aware of, and express his feelings. When the activity occurs in a group, the members have the additional advantage of sharing in others' expressions and of developing fellow-feeling. Increased socialization is another important therapeutic effect nurse-artists/art appreciators seek in the use of art. A corollary benefit is improved communication between the patient and the nurse or between the patient and others.

Obviously, self-knowledge and fellow-feeling are consistent with the aim of humanistic nursing to nurture well-being and more-being. A person develops his human potential and becomes the unique individual he is through his relationships with other men.

NURSING AS ART

Thus far, this chapter has been concerned with the relatedness of nursing and art. It was seen that nurses may study arts and humanities for a broader understanding of the human situation, may express their nursing worlds through various art forms, and may use the arts therapeutically. Now the question is raised whether nursing is an art, and if so, what kind of art.

---

[7] Carol Ann Christoffers, "Movigenic Nursing: An Expanded Dimension," *Humanities and the Arts,* p.95.
[8] Garner, p. 40.
[9] Picasso as quoted in *My Name Is Asher Lev.*
[10] John Hersey, *The Conspiracy* (New York: Alfred A. Knopf, 1972), p. 82.

Artful Application

Even the most scientific nurses do not deny that nursing is, in some way, an art. But precisely how the art and science of nursing are interrelated is not clear. For example, Abdellah writes:

> "The art of nursing must not be confused with the science of nursing. The former concerns itself with intuitive and technical skills (often ritualistic), and also the more supportive aspects of nursing; the latter concerns itself with scientific truths. Both are important. They are interwoven and complement each other."[11]

However, Abdellah gives no further elaboration of this point. Usually, when nurses are asked about the relatedness of the art and the science of nursing, the view expressed is that science has to do with general principles and laws that govern nursing and art has to do with the particular application of principles in individual cases. Furthermore, when a nurse describes some event as "beautiful nursing" and is pressed to elaborate, she usually describes nursing actions that were performed "artfully," "skillfully," "harmoniously." Thus, in some way, the art of nursing has to do with the nurse's response to human needs through actions that are purposeful and aesthetic.

Useful Art

In current usage, the term "art" is most commonly associated with the beautiful, that is, with aesthetics or the fine arts, Frequently, it is restricted even more to signify one group of the fine arts, namely, painting and sculpture. For instance, one refers simply to an "art exhibit" or an "art" museum but specifies further "a center for the performing arts."

However, historically the word "art" was related to utility and knowledge, and its traditional meanings still exist today. For example, we speak of "industrial arts" and "arts and crafts" through which useful things are produced. On the other hand, "liberal arts" (work befitting a free man) are those related to skills of the mind. We also refer to the art of medicine, of teaching, of nursing, of politics, of navigation, of military strategy, and so forth.

The word "art" can refer to both the effect of human work (works of art) and the cause of things produced by human work (the knowledge and skill of the artist). It is obvious that not only knowledge but also some form of work and skill are involved in all art, useful or fine. "Art" is the root of "artisan" as well as of "artist."[12]

Some arts, such as nursing, medicine, and teaching, may be considered useful, yet they differ from other useful arts, such as industrial arts, for they

---

[11] Faye G. Abdellah, "The Nature of Nursing Sceince," *Nursing Research,* Vol. XVIII (September–October, 1969), p. 393.

[12] "Art," *The Great Ideas:* A Syntopicon of Great Books of the Western World I, Vol. 2, 1952, pp. 64-65.

do not result in tangible products. Nursing for instance, aims purposively for well-being, more-being, health, comfort, growth. These are the results of the art of nursing. As an artist, therefore, the nurse must know how to obtain desired effects and must work skillfully to get them. The nurse cannot make well-being or comfort or health as one can make a shoe or a painting or a speech. The art of nursing involves a skillful doing rather than a making. Furthermore, nursing is concerned with changes in human persons not merely with the transformation of physcial objects. It is intersubjective and transactional, so the art of nursing must involve a doing with and a being with.

Performing Art

Along this vein, nursing may be viewed as a kind of performing art. Fahy, nurse-educator-actress, draws an interesting comparison between the process of nursing and acting in a drama.

> "In a play the actors know certain things, there are a certain number of given circumstances: plot, events, epoch, time, and plan of action, conditions of life, director's interpretation. The technical things are also there: setting, props, lights, sound effects, and so forth. But it remains at the time of curtain for the actors to go on alone and produce. In the act of nursing there are some known facts that the nursing student or the nurse can pick up: name, age, religion, ethnic background, medical diagnosis, and plan of care (sometimes), her own background knowledge and experience, and her own unique personality. However, when she encounters other patients—watch it! The same thing happens in the teaching-learning process."

> "Edward A. Wright in *Understanding Today's Theater* says about the actor and acting something which I believe about the nurse and nursing.

> '...the actor...is his own instrument. His tools are himself, his talent, and his ability. Unlike other creative artists, he must work through and with his own body, voice, emotions, appearance, and his own elusive personal quality... He uses his intelligence, his memory of emotions, his experiences, and his knowledge of himself and his fellow men— but always he is his own instrument.' "[13]

Here is another example of viewing nursing as a performing art. Once a nurse was trying to describe the nursing care she received from another nurse when she had been ill. She struggled with some details of finer points and then summed it up by saying, "I felt her nursing care was just like a symphony. That's the only way I can describe it."

These comparisons bring many aesthetic qualities to mind, for instance, harmony, rhythm, tone, feeling. Nursing is like music and drama in other ways. The nursing procedure, like a musical score or a play script, allows for individual interpretations, adaptations, and embellishments. Although nurses follow the same general principles, each can develop her own unique style.

---

[13] Ellen T. Fahy, "Nursing Process as a Performing Art," *Humanities and the Arts,* p. 124.

If nursing really is viewed as a performing art, there are opportunities for creative exploration and development of the art of nursing. And furthermore, these individualized styles of nursing are worthy of description and sharing.

Another similarity is the ephemeral character of nursing, music, and drama. A particular nursing transaction, like a concert or play, is transitory, short-lived. Yet the effects may be long-lasting and remembered. There is this difference in nursing, I believe. Each nursing transaction may flow into a stream of nursing care extending continuously over 24 hours a day for weeks, months, years. And many individual nurses "get into the act." How does this affect the art of nursing? How is nursing like and unlike the other performing arts? The answers to these and similar questions must come from the nurse-artists.

HUMANISTIC NURSING AS CLINICAL ART

The relatedness of nursing and art, viewed existentially, is more basic, more fundamental than mere similarity of qualities and characteristics as discussed above. Both art and nursing are kinds of lived dialogue. In both, man responds to his world of men and things through distance and relation. They affect him and he affects them with the creative force of his relation.

In fact, one may say further that humanistic nursing is *itself* an art—a clinical art—creative and existential. This is evident when one returns again to the thing itself, to the nursing dialogue as it is lived in the everyday world.

In genuine meeting the nurse recognizes the patient as distinct from herself and turns to him as a presence. She is fully present to him, authentically with her whole being and is open to him, not as an object, but as a presence, a human being with potentials. In such a genuine lived dialogue, the nurse sees within the patient a form (that is, a possibility) of well-being or more-being (or comfort or health or growth, and so forth). Like a beautiful landscape inspiring a painter or poet, the form in the patient addresses itself to the nurse, a call for help demanding recognition and response. The form is clearer than experienced objects; it is not an image of her fancy; it exists in the present although it is not "objective." The relation in which the nurse (artist) stands to the form is real for it affects her and she affects it. If she enters into genuine relation with the patient (I-Thou) her effective power (caring, nursing skills, hope) brings forth the form (well-being, more-being, comfort, growth), just as the painter's or poet's power and skill create a painting or a poem.

Of course, there is this difference. The art of nursing, being goal-directed and intersubjective, is more complex than the arts of painting and poetry, for example. As a clinical art, it involves *being with* and *doing with*. For the patient must participate as an active subject to actualize the possibility (form) within himself. Perhaps the art of nursing could be described as transactional. Not only does the nurse see the possibilities in the patient but the patient also sees a form in the nurse (for example, possibility of help, of comfort, of support), and he responds in relation to bring it forth.

Then the question logically may be raised: Is the patient's responses in relation (I-Thou) a necessary condition for the art of nursing? Or to state it differently: can there be any art of nursing the infant, the unresponsive, the comatose, the dying? I would answer that the art of nursing can exist even if the relation is not mutual. For as Buber writes,

> "Even if the man to whom I say *Thou* is not aware of it in the midst of his experience, yet relation may exist. For *Thou* is more than *It* realises. No deception penetrates here; here is the cradle of Real Life."[14]

DIALOGICAL NURSING: ART-SCIENCE

Art and science, like nursing, represent angular views. Each is a view with a particular purpose. They are human responsses to the everyday world in which man lives. Existentially speaking, each is a form of living dialogue between man and his human situation.

It it possible that there is in nursing a kind of human response to reality that is a combination, a true synthesis of art and science? The more one focuses on nursing as it is lived, on the intersubjective transaction as it is experienced in the everyday world, the more questions arise about it as art and science. Elements of both art and science are evident in nursing. The practicing nurse must integrate them in her mode of being in the situation.

While Dr. Josephine Paterson was developing a methodology of inquiry from a clinical nursing process and describing her construct of the "all-at-once," she was so intent on communicating the interrelated reality of the art and science elements in nursing, that she welded them together with a hyphen into one word, "art-science." And even then there is some dissatisfaction when the weld is interpreted merely as a seam. For the combination is more than additive; it is a new synthetic whole.

I experienced a similar difficulty in trying to describe the synthesis of art and science that takes place in the nursing process. The nursing dialogue reflects the orientations of art and science for it involves both the patient's and the nurse's subjective and objective worlds. I believe the synthesis of art and science is *lived* by the nurse in the nursing act. This is a phenomenon more readily experienced than described.

Yet if we truly experience nursing as a kind of art-science, as a particular kind of flowing, synthesizing, subjective–objective intersubjective dialogue, then nursing offers a unique path to human knowledge and it is our responsibility to try to describe and share it.

---

[14] Martin Buber, *I and Thou,* 2nd ed., trans. Ronald Gregor Smith (New York: Charles Scribner's Sons, 1958), p. 9.

9
A HEURISTIC CULMINATION

This chapter presents an application of the humanistic nursing practice theory over time and an outcome. The outcome represents my present conscious conceptualization of my personal theory of nursing. It has grown out of my nursing practice experience, my reflecting, relating, describing, and synthesizing. This is heuristic culmination of much mulling over my lived world of nursing.

ANGULAR VIEW: PRESENT PERSPECTIVE

In 1971 after a presentation on concept development I heard myself in a chatty response to the audience declare my unique theory of nursing. It was based in constructs that I had developed and conceptualized. Previously I had viewed these constructs only as distinct entities. My synthesis of them surprised me. This was the first time I conveyed them as my why, how, and what of nursing. This synthesis may have emerged as a sequence to my reexamination and reflection on each of these constructs in preparation for this 1971 presentation.[1] Now it became evident that their sequential evolvement had a logic that had come from my being without my awareness.

Since 1971 I have planned to reflect on these synthetic constructs to better understand how they relate to one another complementarily. Why? To further the development of these constructs and to state them as propositions. Statements of propositions are movement toward nursing theory. Theory is considered here as a conceptualized vision teased out of my knowing from my nursing experience.

---

[1] Josephine G. Paterson, "A Perspective on Teaching Nursing: How Concepts Become," in *A Conceptual Approach to the Teaching of Nursing in Baccalaureate Programs,* a report of a project directed by Rose M. Herrera (Washington, D.C.: The Catholic University of America, School of Nursing, 1973), pp. 17-27.

Like Elie Wiesel, the novelist and literary artist, I write to better understand and to attest to happenings. This chapter is the fruit of this endeavor.

The first term, "comfort," was developed as a construct in 1967. After recording and exploring my clinical experiential data, a conceptualized response emerged to my question: "Why, as a nurse, am I in the clinical health-nursing situation?" The second term, "clinical," was developed as a construct in 1968. It was a conceptualized response to a dialectical process within myself. I asked, "What is clinical?" I answered, "I am a clinician." I asked, "As a nurse clinician what do I do; what is the condition of my being in the nursing situation?" I answered, "This described would equate to clinical." Consequently I compared and contrasted two nursing experiences similarly labeled to properly grasp the principle of "clinical" for conceptualization. The third term or phrase, "all-at-once," arose intuitively within me as a construct in 1969 and was partially conceptualized. It arose after mulling over other nurses' published clinical data and asking, "What can you tell me of the clinical nursing situation?" "What do you perceive as the nature of nursing?" Therese G. Muller's, Ruth Gilbert's and my thought on the nursing situation merged into a view of these as multifariously loaded with all levels of incomparable data, the "all-at-once." Incommensurables relate to the nature of nursing and its concerns. How can one study unrelated appearances? Muller often used an historical approach while Gilbert emphasized individualization. In humanistic nursing practice theory a descriptive, intersubjective, phenomenological approach is proposed for greater understanding and attestation of the events and process of the nursing situation. The construction of "comfort, clinical, and all-at-once" I would now label as conceptualized phenomenologically. I view them as relevant phenomena to any nurse and this nurse-in-her-nursing-world.

Theory: Unrest, Beginning Involvement

This desire to develop nursing theory goes back to my years (1959-64) as a faculty member in a graduate nursing program. I fussed with the idea, did not know exactly what I was fussing about, and expressed my desire, interest, and concern poorly. Much, I am sure now, to others' dismay. Teaching in nursing was an offering of multitudinous theories developed in and for other disciplines using nursing examples. There were both similarities and differences in the many nursing examples in which attempts were made to describe the qualities of the participants' beings. Emphasis was placed on the observations by the nurse of the others' responses in the nursing situation. Nursing education was rife with lengthy repetitive examples utilized to focus on particular variations. I desired a unifying base applicable to all nursing situations. This was not a seeking for conformity nor an attempt to negate individuality. Certainly I did not want such a base to exclude individual nurses' talents. Rather this base, foundation of nursing indicative of the nature of nursing, would heuristically promote endless variations to flow, blossom, cross-pollinate, and evolve.

In these observations and thinkings I was attempting to understand, sort out, and clarify the questions that underlay my puzzlement. This puzzlement arose out of my 18 years in nursing practice and education. In a theory course and a philosophy of science course, while in doctoral study, I recognized and learned to label my unrest and puzzlement as a recognition of the need for nusring theory.

In 1966 in discussing my purposes for doctoral study, I expressed this unrest and puzzlement. I viewed my varied past experiences in nursing as excellent. I sought time to reflect on the past 24 years of living nursing to see what it could tell me, and to come to better understand its meaning to the profession of nursing. The philosophical nature of these questions and what they express of myself is evident. Such personal revelation at this time is no risk, and withholding would only deprive myself and others of the answers that might be brought forth.

As in most school situations initially responding to class assignments and involvement in new clinical situations consumed my time and thwarted my personal, professional interests. When I commented on this my interests were interpreted to me as a desire to live in the past. Living in the present was recommended and terms like "up-to-date" and "progressive" were employed. I felt stopped cold. I had never veiwed myself as old fashioned or non-progressive. Many of my past nursing experiences were still avant-garde as compared with general current practices.

There was something different though in recalling and reflecting on the past as opposed to current experiences. One's past would be visible in view of how one approached and experienced the present. Self-confrontation moved me beyond confining myself either to the past or to the present. In my writings one could detect a comparison of what had been known with what was coming to be known. It was as if a light of a different hue lit up the whole—past and present—as a different scene. Similariy I viewed and experienced my clinical experience differently. I gained awareness of a quality of my being that always had been there, but which I hid. Now I valued this part, struggled with it, and expressed it directly with courage, integrity, and pride. The power with which this self-actualization imbued me has been sculpturing my "I" into a form of my choosing ever more acceptable to me, and accepting of others.

Concept Development

In a nursing theory course the final assignment was: develop a concept relevant to nursing. Again I found myself struggling. The didactically stated importance of investing precious time and energy into constructing a synthetic conceptualization of a term eluded me. Time and energy spent to better understand man as he was known to me in the nursing situation seemed so limited. In these situations persons were expressing so many things at one time, how could the conceptualization of one term be relevant. Finally I understood: no one was saying that any one term could equate any particular or group of nursing situations. They were saying that to communicate the nature or experience of nursing with words, to develop nursing theory, relevant terms needed clarification as to the meaning they conveyed and delineation as to their inclusiveness and exclusiveness.

As this struggle subsided I could hear, "a term could be developed as a concept or synthetic construct if one conceptualized its why, what, how, when, and where and how these interrelated." In approaching concept development the last but not least hurdle was, what term did I consider relevant enough in nursing to expend this precious time and energy on considering the many possibilities. The first term I began to intellectually play with was "ambivalence." Now, I would attribute my selection of "ambivalence" to my then existing ambivalence about conceptualizing a synthetic construct. Then, I based its selection only on its existence in my clinical nursing world. I was working therapeutically on a regular, individual basis with an ambivalent adolescent male labeled diagnostically as a paranoid schizophrenic. I began to consider my clinically recorded data of my sessions with Bob through ambivalence. What were the relationships between why, how, what, when, and where Bob expressed ambivalence?

Struggling with the term "ambivalence" involved and interested me in concept development. During this phase I overcame my fear of exposing my thoughts, I took the risk, and my courage had the upper hand. Nevertheless, another choice had to be made since now I was not willing to invest this much time on conceptualizing "ambivalence" as so relevant to nursing. Perhaps this signified that my own ambivalence had dissipated. And again, I faced the question, what term would I want to develop as a synthetic construct?

The next question that occurred to me was, what term would indicate why, as a nurse, I am in the clinical health-nursing situation? Did I view my value mainly as growth, health, freedom, or openness promotion? I worked for a while with each of these terms and eventually discarded them. Some long-hospitalized persons with whom I was working on a demonstration psychiatric unit to prepare them for a more independent and appropriate form of community living would never be stably balanced in health, growing, freedom or openness. For many, these could be only flitting memorable beautiful moments. Still I believed I was very much there in the nursing situation for these persons, as well as for those who moved into the community and found work and social satisfactions. Something occurred between all of these 15 patients and myself—and that was nursing.

COMFORT:WHY

While considering what construct to conceptualize, I was in the process of recording my three-hour, twice a week interactions in the demonstration unit. I reflected on these interactions and waited for the data to reveal to me the major value underlying my nursing practice. Then the term "comfort" came to mind. Perhaps at this point I became comfortable in this unit, or perhaps the unit, itself, became a more comfortable setting. When I had first begun my experience with this demonstration unit, it was still being planned and the hospital was new to me. However, the term "comfort" has long been associated with nursing. One can find it as a historical constant throughout the professional nursing literature. The term had been used recently in an ANA publication.[2] When I considered the idea of comforting in nursing practice I felt such experiences had fulfilled and satisfied me, made me feel adequate. I could recall specific experiences that went back to my initial nursing practice settings. I could conceive of comfort as an umbrella under which all the other terms—growth, health, freedom, and openness—could be sheltered. Some of my contemporaries scoffed and viewed this term as much too trivial.

Now, again reviewing my months of gathered clinical data, I sorted out 12 nurse behaviors that I viewed as aiming toward patient comfort. They were:

1. I focused on recognizing patients by name, being certain I was correct about their names, and using their names often and appropriately. I also introduced myself. Names were viewed as supportive to the internalization of personal identification, dignity, and worth.

2. I interpreted, taught, and gave as much honest information as I could about patients' situations when it was sought or when puzzlement was apparent. This was based in the belief that it was their life, and choice was their prerogative as they were their own projects.

3. I verbalized my acceptance of patients' expressions of feeling with explanations of why I experienced these feelings of acceptance when I could do this authentically and appropriately.

4. When verbalizations of acceptance were not appropriate, I acted out this acceptance by staying with or doing for when appropriate.

5. I expressed purposely, to burst asunder negative self-concepts, my authentic human tender feelings for patients when appropriate and acceptable.

6. I supported patients' rights to agape-type love relationships with others: families, other staff, and other patients.

7. I showed respect for patients as persons with the right to make as many choices for themselves as their current capabilities allowed.

8. I attempted to help patients consider their currently expressed feelings and behaviors in light of past life experiences and patterns, like and unlike their current ones.

---

[2] American Nurses' Association, Division on Psychiatric-Mental Health Nursing, *Statement on Psychiatric Nursing Practice* (New York: American Nurses' Association, 1967), p. IV.

9. I encouraged patients' expression to better understand their behavioral messages and to enable me to respond overtly as therapeutically as possible.

10. I verified my intuitive grasp of how patients were experiencing events by questions and comments and being alert to their responses.

11. I attempted to encourage hope realistically through discussing individual therapeutic gains that could be derived from patients' investment in therapeutic opportunties available to them.

12. I supported appropriate patient self-images with as many concrete "hard to denies" as possible.

Each of these nurse behaviors was repeatedly evident in the months of recording patient-nurse interactions. For the conceptualization of the term "comfort," a representative clinical example was given to enhance the meaning of the behavior cited (see Appendix). When compiling materials for the conceptualization of this term, I found 12 assumptions about psychiatric nursing that I had written for the theory course in one of the first class sessions. Although these assumptions were expressed in different words, their congruence with my 12 selected behaviors made me believe that these behaviors were somehow verified both in my conceptualized philosophy of psychiatric nursing and in my behavior while being a psychiatric nurse.

Next I struggled with an idealistic conception of comfort as opposed to a continuum of behavior which would indicate a person's degree or state of discomfort–comfort. Again, reflecting on and teasing out aspects of my data, I set up four behaviorally recognizable criteria for estimating a person's discomfort–comfort state:

1. Relationships with other persons which confirm one as an existent important person.

2. Affective adaptation to the environment in accord with knowledge, potential, and values.

3. Awareness of and response to the reality of the now with understanding of the influence of and separation from the past.

4. Appreciation and recognition of both powers and limitations which enlighten the alternatives of the future.

These behavioral criteria, too, could each be spread on a continuum to evaluate the effects of this aim of nursing on a patient's actual comfort status at any particular point in time.

Considering the concept of comfort as a proper aim of psychiatric nursing brought forth the necessity of considering its opposite, discomfort, as a concept. Evidence for the existence of discomfort could be inferred in the absence of the above behavioral criteria.

The basic foundation to justify the concept of comfort as a proper aim of psychiatric nursing would be both organic and environmental. In our culture, among the species man, we are moving toward being able to effect some organic conditions by genetic controls and surgical and chemical means. The professions have struggled long years to influence environmental deterrents to comfort. If an individual as a fetus, or as an infant, or young child never internalizes comfort of any kind from his environs, the probability of initiating a continuum within himself as an adult that is propelled toward comfort seems unlikely. Such individuals, lacking any potential capacity for comfort, I suspect are rare. There is evidence for the existence of this dormant seed of comfort in persons with schizophrenia in the hospital setting. Consider how repetitively and ambivalently they "reach out" to authority figures. This dormant comfort seed requires nourishment of a high quality for testing whether it can develop and bear the fruits of health, growth, freedom, and openness.

When the development of this synthetic construct of comfort was discussed in the theory course a question was raised: Is a person who denies all feeling, presents himself as emotionally dead, comfortable? If feelings are not relegated to the mind alone, as the effects of a peptic ulcer cannot be relegated to the stomach, if feelings are an essential of the nature of humanness, a human who denies this essential of his nature would not fit into this concept as comfortable. This synthetic construct of comfort, like its synonym contentment, described by Plutarch A.D. 46-120, does not imply passivity, resignation, retirement, or a simple avoiding of trouble. Plutarch said, "Contentment comes very dear if its price is inactivity."[3] I would perceive of comfort or contentment as implying that a human being was all he could be in accordance with his potential at any particular time in any particular situation.

Continuing the aforementioned twelve nurse behaviors, observing behavior through the four established criteria and conceptualizing the construct of comfort, I began to wonder. Was I seeing what I had decided was the state of psychiatric patients' conditions of being? Was I projecting discomfort onto patients? I did not expect straight answers. Nonetheless, I decided to ask patients about their discomfort-comfort states to verify my perception of the condition of their beings. All fourteen patients I asked assured me by their responses that I was not projecting or seeing discomfort where it did not exist.

Some described physical discomfort and sought the cause within and outside themselves (either another caused it, or another could cure it, pills would cure it), negatively viewed self-images, guilt based in their behaviors or thoughts. One patient defined comfort by analogy and stated directly to my surprise that he seldom felt comfortable and that his excessive ritualistic behavior was his way of coping with his discomfort. One repetitively stated a happy illusion that he seemed to hang on to for dear life. When I asked what he would do if this illusion was not truth, he said that he had never considered

---

[3] Plutarch, "Contentment," in *Gateway to the Great Books,* Vol. 10, *Philosophical Essays* (Chicago: Encyclopaedia Britannica, 1963), p. 265.

this possibility. I knew he had been confronted with the truth of his situation many times in many ways. One patient merely looked directly at me and walked away. Then I again reviewed my clinical recorded data to see what kinds of knowledge nursing with an aim to comfort would infer as necessary. Fifty-two items of knowledge were extrapolated from the clinical examples selected as representative of the twelve nurse behaviors. These items were categorized under broad cognitive and affective domains. This was an arbitrary point of separation. They were teased apart simply as an aid to conceptualization and understanding. If these knowledge domains had related to one another in a simple direct manner, I would have conveyed them in a table in which each would have been across from its mate. Their relationships to one another were far too complex to be handled in any such a way. The affective domain knowledge areas were a dynamic internalized synthesis of several knowledge areas from the cognitive domain. Thus, the expression of these affective knowledge areas was evidence of the practice of nursing as an artful form of expressing cognitive knowing.

In looking directly at the discomfort of long-term hospitalized psychiatric patients, I found myself faced with behaviors that resulted possibly from a muddle of many contributaries. What in the behavior resulted from lifetime environmental influences and compounded responses that deepened scars? What resulted from long-term hospitalization? How many varieties of ills superimposed like layers on the above were expressed in what I saw as discomfort in these psychiatric patients? Diagnostic classifications are necesary for statistical economic planning reasons. Still, how naively and superficially they convey the human therapeutic care needs of each person.

At this point of construct development I saw a positive relationship in my thinking about comfort as a proper aim of psychiatric nursing and Viktor Frankl's description of his aim in logotherapy toward meaning. I had struggled with the idea of aiming at comfort while with patients who possessed ability and a favorable prognosis, often purposefully and deliberately asking them to consider ideas that caused them immediate greater discomfort. Frankl's quotes from Nietzsche and Geothe supported my altruistic intention. Nietzsche said:

"He who has a why to live can bear almost any how."[4]

Goethe said:

"When we take man as he is, we make him worse; but when we take man as if he were already what he should be, we promote him to what he can be."[5]

In conclusion to this stage of development of a synthetic construct of comfort as an aim of psychiatric nursing I can say: Comfort is an aim toward

---

[4] Viktor E. Frankl, *From Death-Camp to Existentialism* (Boston: Beacon Press, 1961), p. 103.
[5] *Ibid.*, p. 110.

which persons' conditions of being move through relationship with others by internalizing freedom from painful controlling effects of the past. These effects have inhibited their self-control, realistic planning, and prevented them from being all that they could be in accordance with their potential at any particular time in any particular situation. I would project this as an aim for nursing in all situations although the data for constructing this conceptualization were gathered in a clinical psychiatric setting.

CLINICAL: HOW

As a component of my doctoral examinations I was faced with having to rewrite a clinical paper. This led to my deliberately and personally choosing to conceptualize a synthetic construct of "clinical." This was my decision. It speaks well for the value of having had the experience of conceptualizing "comfort." Often it is said that man repeats that which he finds as meaningful and good. This choice also signifies a real overcoming of my resistance and ambivalence toward synthetic construct development in a year's time.

"Clinical" was developed as a synthetic construct in 1968. It was a conceptualized response to a dialectical process within myself. If I am a clinician, then "how" I am in the health-nursing situation would equate to "clinical." In conceptualizing this construct I teased out of my lived-nursing-world the "how" of my working toward my own and others' comfort.

Confusion, over what was meant when persons casually and currently popularly attributed the term "clinical" to situations and persons, called forth this conceptualization. It grew out of comparing and contrasting two nursing consultation experiences in the psychiatric-mental health area. Beginning this conceptualization I would have referred to both these experiences as "clinical." At the termination of the conceptualization they were both "clinical." They were very different experiences for me, and yet of equal value in my advancement toward my more of being. Prior to this conceptualization because my attending emotions were so disturbing and unacceptable to me in relation to one of these experiences, automatically I repressed part of them and found reasons to suppress the rest of them. Unfortunately, all else that was of value to me in having lived this experience was integrally enmeshed with these emotions. This, too, became unavailable to my conscious awareness. Conceptualization made recall and reflection a necessity. Clinical includes inherently a process of experiencing awarely and then recalling, looking at, reflecting on, and sorting out to come to knowing.

Before knowing how to approach the rewriting of my clinical paper as a partial requirement for receiving my doctoral degree I experienced a depression. I felt frightened, angry, and inadequate. The original clinical paper had been judged as more intellectual and scholarly than clinical. I could conceive of only two alternatives. Both seemed self-defeating. One, I could revise my former clinical paper into a more intellectual and scholarly paper that still would not be clinical and would still leave my "I" out. Or, two, I could revise my former clinical paper, dump all my feelings in the situational experience, blame everyone else for these feelings, and culminate at least with my clinical passions visible. Conflict resulted from my considering pursuing either of these routes. I was immobilized for a time. A time limitation and time passing pushed me to begin somewhere. I began. Choosing the second alternative in the belief that at least through writing I would better understand what I had lived in the experience.

I could support the value of dredging up these old feelings and looking at them. Authentically letting myself be aware of what I had experienced, not necessarily communicating this or acting out in accordance with these redredged feelings; just really looking at them might allow me choice in how I wanted to live with them. One support for the value of looking at these old feelings was my own past three and one-half years in psychoanalysis in which I profited through such a process. The other support was my readings of the past two years. These included works of Russell, [6] Nietzsche,[7] Plato,[8] Popper,[9] Dewey,[10] Buber,[11], Bergson,[12] Cousins,[13] and de Chardin.[14]

As this experience became in shape and meaning through my writing, I began to view this product as like an existential play filled with blatant atrocities and absurdities that had to be nonrealities. This production, also, made visible beautiful raw data. As meaning in this clinical nursing consultation experience as a graduate student became evident, comparision of it with the meaning of clinical work experiences in nursing consultation situations flowed naturally. Then joy, it was like sunshine burst forth and warmed my spirit.

Before entering school, I was, for two years, a mental health psychiatric clinical nurse consultant to a staff of forty-five visiting nurses. I had become intrigued

---

[6] Bertrand Russell, *The Autobiography of Bertrand Russell* (Boston: Little, Brown and Company, 1968) and *An Outline of Philosophy* (Cleveland: The World Publishing Company, 1967).

[7] Frederick Nietzsche, "Beyond Good and Evil," trans. Helen Zimmern, in *The Philosophy of Nietzsche* (New York: The Modern Library, 1927) and "Thus Spake Zarathustra," trans. Thomas Common, in *The Philosophy of Nietzsche* (New York: The Modern Library, 1927).

[8] Plato, *The Republic,* trans. Francis MacDonald Cornford (New York, Oxford University Press, 1945).

[9] Karl Popper, *Conjectures and Refutations* (New York: Basic Books, Pbulishers, 1963).

[10] John Dewey, *The Knowing and the Known* (Boston: The Beacon Press, 1949) and "The Process of Thought from How We Think," in *Gateway to the Great Books,* ed. Robert W. Hutchins, et al. (Chicago: Encyclopaedia Britannica, 1963).

[11] Martin Buber, *Between Man and Man,* trans. Ronald Gregor Smith (Boston: Beacon Press, 1955); *I and Thou,* 2nd ed., trans. Ronald Gregor Smith (New York: Charles Scribner's Sons, 1958); *The Knowledge of Man,* ed. Maurice Friedman (New York: Harper & Row, Publishers, 1965).

[12] Henri Bergson, "Introduction to Metaphysics," in *Philosophy in the Twentieth Century,* Vol. III, ed. William Barrett and Henry D. Aiken (New York: Random House, 1962) and "Time in the History of Western Philosophy," in *Philosophy in the Twentieth Century,* Vol. III, ed. William Barrett and Henry D. Aiken (New York: Random House, 1962).

[13] Norman Cousins, *Who Speaks for Man* (New York: The Macmillan Company, 1953).

[14] Pierre Teilhard de Chardin, *Letters from a Traveler,* (New York: Harper & Row, Publishers, 1962) and *The Phenomenon of Man* (New York: Harper Torchbooks, Harper & Row, Publishers, 1961).

with what I had come to understand about consultation related to clinical situations. I wrote a paper for publication on the subject. Busy in the process of returning to school, and awaiting the publication of two other papers—both of these proceedings feeling unreal and out of my control, not to mention self-exposing—I merely filed in my desk the typed submittable rendition of this consultation paper. Now, I dug it out. This meant that I had two conceptualized presentations of similar type personal experiences in nursing consultation to compare and contrast. From these, my conceptualization of clinical, and the values on which my clinical practice rests, could be extrapolated.

A Student Consultation Experience Becomes Clinical

In the graduate student nurse consultation experience I felt helpless, confused, unwanted, guilty, anxious, and unimportant. It was a passion-filled experience for me. As a nurse-student consultant among interdisciplinary nonstudent-consultants I experienced dependency for my being and doing on persons I viewed as anxious, critical, nonempathetic, and inadequate. We were attempting to offer consultation to a professional group of nonpsychiatric mental health oriented consultees who were anxious and felt inadequate in this area. I felt forced into an observer rather than participant mode of being, and my recorded data support this. Impotency comes to mind when I recall this experience, as well as a racking rage and suffering that obliterates feelings of love, good-will, tenderness, or hope. About that time I was reading Nietzsche's eternal recurrence phenomenon[15] and viewed it most pessimistically— all was awful, it would continue to be awful, life was just a vicious cycle of awfulness.

Defense or health, it is questionable. Suddenly, perhaps it was having hit feelings of rock bottom, I began to view Nietzsche's eternal recurrence phenomenon optimistically. Did the polarization of my negative feelings magnetically call forth my opposite feelings? All, now, contained the new, it would continue to contain the new, life was a series of similar and yet different cycles that always contained the new.

Now my reflections let in hope, positiveness, comradeship, good feelings, and progress made by myself and others in our year and a half together as consultants. During this period we met with the consultees for an hour once or twice a week. The group had continued over this period despite its components of psychiatric mental health professionals and nonpsychiatric mental health profession culturally, professionally, and historically having been quite alienated from one another. Attendance had improved some over time. Toward the end of the year and a half, during the last three months, the focus of discussion was on patients and their worlds for longer periods of time. There was less defensive acting out in which things, fees, time, and mechanics consumed the hour.

---

[15] Nietzsche, *The Philosophy of Nietzsche,* p. 441.

Toward the end of these sessions the consultant chief found more acceptable space in which to meet for the consultation. Eating lunch became part of the session. Food can be looked at in many ways. In this case it seemed to be a cohesive force, rather than a distracting, socializing force. Was this because of the underlying meanings food had for these people? Or was the meaning of food in this situation concrete? Now the consultees could have their lunch served to them while receiving consultation. This latter saved their time and meant money to them. This was a giving gesture on the part of the consultants even though the lunch monies did come out of the project funding source. The meaning of food was never discussed in the group. I wonder if this feeding was done with deliberate awareness or was just serendipitous.

During the last three months of meeting I began to feel related on a deeper level with a few of the participants, consultants and consultees. Individual to individual we began to communicate collaboratively with one another as professional colleagues. We discussed both patients' lived worlds and the meaning of psychiatric mental health terms and ideas. I can conceive, now, that this may have occurred between other group members before or after sessions. Initially there were often only two to three consultees to five or six consultants. Later the total group containted fifteen to sixteen people. Now I would project that the very existence of this group could influence future groups positively.

A Clinical Work Consultation Experience

In this work consultation experience my feelings were openness, reflectiveness, pain, helpfulness, alertness, searchfulness, appreciativeness, receptiveness, responsiveness, wantedness, competence, joy, and importance. It was both a passionate and a dispassionate experience. As a working consultant I met with consultees either alone or as part of a collaborating team of consultants. Often the situations the consultees presented which they struggled with and stayed in struck me with awe. They aroused my humility while making me feel whole and fulfilled in my participation with the consultees. In my explorations of and with the consultees my presence, thereness, and authenticity were all important. Buber would say that my aim in consultation was to "imagine the real" of what the consultee and the patients and families she discussed with me "could be."[16] This was my initial disposition. I aimed to be open to and accept the potentials of these others.

In initial receptiveness, grounded in my comfort, was the "key" to the "door" of the consultant-consultee "I-Thou" relation in which I could come to know intuitively the experience of this particular other nurse-in-her-lived-nursing-world. The consultees offered their lived-nursing-worlds each in their unique ways. Some discussed directly their pains, joys, adequacies, and inadequacies. Some discussed indirectly their panic, success, action, and immobilization. Some beyond being able to discuss their lived-worlds

---

[16] Buber, *The Knowledge of Man,* Appendix, p. 168.

spontaneously acted out their lived-worlds. For example, these often behaved toward me as their patients and families behaved toward them. These kinds of acted out lived-worlds I had to sense my way into to understand. When I began to wonder what it was that they wanted from consultation to take back to their lived-nursing-worlds, I would pull out of the "I-Thou" form of relating. This wonderment became my conscious clue. It was time to reflect and look at what my explorations had uncovered.

At this point transcending this "I-Thou" relation, I would look at "It." Seeing, now, what was within me, what the condition of my being was that I had intuitively taken on from the consultee, I would set it apart from myself, and see it as an empathic response. I knew that these feelings I experienced which I received existentially, globally through the compound of the consultee's words, tone inflection, volume, facial expression, posture, and positioning to me were what she experienced in her-nursing world. Verbalization of this empathized understanding fulfilled several purposes: (1) it conveyed my sympathy or joy with, and always my caring, (2) it validated that I saw it as it was for this nurse, and (3) it opened the door to our working through the possible meanings of the nurse's experience and to speculating about outcomes of alternative future nurse actions and behaviors.

Cognitively the range of these consultation discussions was broad. Some common themes were social and health histories of families, pertinent psychological growth and development factors of persons in the families of concern to the consultees, relationships between persons within the situations, resources available to the families, ways the consultees could relate with the parents and patients' families, friends, and other professionals in the situation, and the meaning of all these themes to the particular consultee.

This clinical consultation experience necessitated my being certain ways. It necessitated my being authentic with myself with regard to what responses were called forth in me in relating with a particular consultee. I viewed honesty with the consultee as a value necessary to the consultation process. In approaching the consultation I needed to be open to the consultee's angular view and predisposed toward an "I-Thou" relationship. The "I-Thou" relating necessitated subsequent scientific understanding extrapolated from it through reflection on it as "I-It." My hope in consultation was to offer both a cognitive, as well as, an ontic experience in which a mutual feeling apart from and toward the other would exist. This latter seemed most important to me. If the consultee experienced my being authentically present with her, she then would be apt to offer this type of relationship to the patients and families of concern to her.

Results of Comparison

The two clinical consultation experiences were juxtaposed, contrasted, questioned, related, and synthesized to envision their unified contribution to the construct of "clinical." The synthetic construct of "clinical" is not viewed as a mere juxtaposing, a disintegrating, or reconstructing of the contributions to my knowing from either of these experiences. This comparison is viewed as a facing of the multiplicities they both present. The synthesis is an illumination of both experiences with each transfigured through their mutual presence in the "knowing place" of the comparer.[17]

In this comparison my appreciation grew of how I had uniquely implemented and conceptualized clinical consultation in my work experience. I recognized through the comparison that adequate clinical consultation demands both a passionate and dispassionate phase of "I-Thou" and "I-It" relating. Without either of these forms of consultant being-in-the-situation we degrade the term "clinical" if we employ it. Consultation lends itself naturally to a collaborative cooperative relationship. The consultant is dependent on the consultee for presentation of the specifics of particular situations. The consultee is dependent on the consultant for the tailoring of general knowledge to the consultees' particular situations. The relationship if appropriately called consultation is then of necessity interdependent. In being separate from the other while feeling with the other the consultant does not lose the ability to question. Passion undealt with or identification with the consultee inhibits the clinical purpose of the consultant and of the consultation. In identification one feels as if he were the other, rather than turning to the other and feeling with him. The degree of anxiety this provokes in the consultant can prevent looking at the consultation situation and issues in an "I-It" manner. The consultant loses the ability to question.

Through this comparison I was able to reflect on the graduate student nursing consultation experience in an "I-It" way. At this time it became a "clinical" experience for me. The lack of this reflective phase in this experience highlighted the reflective phase already existent in the working clinical consultation experience. The existence of this phase in the working clinical consultation experience highlighted its absence in the graduate student nursing consultation experience. My commonplace nursing world through this comparison became awarely meaningful and availed itself for conceptualization. A situation is not a "clinical" experience until the "would be" clinician can reflect, analyze, categorize, and synthesize it.

Clinical Is

A potentially clinical psychiatric mental health situation becomes "clinical" if the clinician relates to the helpee to awaken his unique potential or ontic wholeness, and noetically transcending this relating conceptualizes its meaning.

Clinician signifies a particular mode of being and a particular kind of cognitive knowledge. With all his human capacity the clinician relates with his clinical-world consciously and deliberately in "I-Thou," and "I-It."

Relating in "I-Thou" with the other in-his-clinical-world the clinician gives himself and receives back the other and himself in the sphere of "the between."

---

[17] Wilfrid Desan, *Planetary Man* (New York: The Macmillan Company, 1972), p. 77.

He knows the other and the more of himself in this relating. He is confirmed and confirms the other through the other's presence with him. Thus, he calls forth the other's actualizing of self through the clinical relationship. In accepting the other as he is the clinician imagines and responds to the reality of his potential for becoming, becoming according to his unique capacity for humanness.

Relating in "I-It" with his clinical world the clinician noetically transcends himself, objectifies himself, and studies his "I-Thou" knowing. He teases it apart. He classifies and studies it. He asks it questions. He compares and contrasts it to other clinical experiences. He discusses its many aspects in dialogue with his "inward," and possibly "outward" "Thous." He reorders its parts. He shapes, creates, plans from and for its clinical existence. Thus, he ever augments a world of heuristic knowing.

This "how" allows the clinical fulfillment of my nursing "why." Comfort is "why" I, as a nurse, am in the health–nursing situation. As conceptualized "comfort" is being able to freely control and plan for one's self, being fully in accord at a particular time, in a particular situation, with one's unique potential. Now, "what" is the nature of the nurse's world, the health–nursing situation?

ALL-AT-ONCE: WHAT

The term "all-at-once," arose within me as a construct that would metaphorically describe the multifarious multiplicities that exist within nursing situations. Completing my comparison of Gilbert's and Muller's written works to grasp how they viewed the nature of psychiatric mental health nursing I found myself mulling over and fussing.[18] Your question is probably, mulling and fussing over what? While I mulled over and fussed I believe I, too, was perplexed. Why was I unsatisfied?

I had compared Gilbert's and Muller's writing styles, their conceptions of man, approaches to nursing, nursing education, supervision, and consultation. Their similarities and differences were noted, and how each presented herself predominantly. Then I cited the nursing communities they sought to influence and those in which they were while writing. Through reviewing their bibliographies and biographies I indicated the sources that had influenced them.

Still I mulled over, fussed, and was perplexed. I awakened in the middle of one night in 1969 understanding what had been causing my struggle. The "all-at-once" was my answer.

The description of single constructs and single examples originally had felt unrelated to the reality of the nurse's world. They oversimplified its complexity. The nature of nursing was complex. It seemed to me that we needed, as a profession, constructs that simplified and allowed clear communications. We, also, needed constructs that conveyed the reality and complexity of the

---

[18] Josephine G. Paterson, "Echo into Tomorrow: A Mental Health Psychiatric Philosophical Conceptualization of Nursing" (D.N.Sc. dissertation, Boston University, 1969).

worlds in which nurses nursed. Perhaps a description of what "all-at-once" expressed for me would convey to others the lived-unobservable-worlds of nurses.

Nurses relate to other man in situations of "all-at-once." The "all-at-once" is equated by me to Buber's "I-Thou" and "I-It" occurring simultaneously and not only in sequence as he expressed it. These two ways that man can relate to and come to know his world and himself demand sequential expression for clear communication. However, the responsible authentic nurse in the nursing arena lives them "all-at-once." Aware of the multifarious multiplicities of her responses to another and at once to the surrounding field of action, the nurse selects and overtly expresses her responses that actualize the purpose, values, and potential of the artful science of professional nursing.

Awareness of the multifarious multiplicities affecting the other and the self in the nursing arena is a component of "I-Thou" relating. Selectively overtly expressing concordantly with the purpose, values, and potential of nursing necessitates a looking at, which is a component of "I-It" relating, while acting and being. Therefore both "I-Thou and I-It" modes of being are "all-at-once."

This necessity for a nurse' duality in her mode of being came to my awareness through comparing Gilbert' and Muller's works, studying Buber's conceptions of man, and considering them in relation to my current and past lived-experiences in the nursing -arena. In my nursing world of "I-Thou" relating reflection is called forth prior to my overt response to allow response selection concordant with my nursing purpose. The very character of multifarious multiplicities of the nursing world undoubtedly has called for nurses to develop their human capacity for duality in their mode of being.

To make these "multifarious multiplicities" explicit I would like to offer a description of a recent, personal nursing experience. In a community psychiatric mental health psychosocial clinic, I sat across from and focused on relating with a psychiatric client. After long years of hospitalization he was now living in a community foster home and visiting the clinic three days a week. When there was no special clinic activity in progress and often even when there was, he sat by himself and played poker. He told me about his game many times, over weeks and months. He dealt out five poker hands. Each hand was dealt to a member of his family, long dead. He did not accept their deadness. One day while describing the poker games and his relatives, he intermittently expressed his fantasies which he projected on to a sweet cheerful 65-year-old community volunteer. She was somewhat deaf. His fantasies were angry. When he gestured toward her, she in a motherly way came over to him, put her arm around him, and her ear down to his mouth. It was a moment of possible client explosion. With my eyes I attempted to communicate with her. This, and the tone of the patient's voice warned her to move away. While this was occurring another patient jealous of my attentions to this patient walked up and down, and in passing negatively commented on the religious background of the man I was sitting with. In the rear of the room a dietician was conducting a group on obesity. And all of this was set to the melodious, sanguine strains of "If I Loved You" being poorly beat out on a piano about ten feet away by another volunteer accompanied in song by a few clients. Meanwhile two staff nurses were observing my part in all this since I was labeled "expert." The client did support me that day and responded to my staying with him. Much to my surprise he began playing poker with me. He dealt me out a hand. This was, at this time, a new behavior on his part. It was movement toward his potential for relating to live persons in his current world. This, again, is just one example of the multifarious multiplicities of one very common type of nursing situation.

The inference from the above is that professional artistic-scientific nurses relate in "I-Thou, I-It, all-at-once" to the specific general, critical nonconsequential, and the healthy ill. This presents a paradoxical dilemma. Nurses, as human beings, have a highly developed capacity for living "all-at-once" in and with the flow of the multifarious multiplicities of their worlds. Nurses, as human beings, like all other human beings, are limited to thinking, interpreting, and expressing conceptually only in succession.

This metaphoric synthetic construct, "all-at-once," has allowed me to better convey how I experience the health nursing situation. It also has aided my understanding of the multifarious multiplicity of angular views expressed by several professionals in responding to and describing a similar situation. I can accept each description as truth for each responder. Each responds with his uniqueness in the situation. Comparing, contrasting, and complementarily synthesizing these multiple views inclusive of their inconsistencies and contradictions, none negating the other, allows a better understanding of man-in-his-world in the health situation than the so frequently presented oversimplifications. These oversimplified presentations usually deal only with what is occurring that is important to the particular interests of the reporter. And they are offered only after the selected material has been put through a process of interpretation and logical sequencing to emphasize the reporter's particular point. In such reporting the existent in the situation labeled unimportant, unacceptable, or unrelated is not considered. Such existents, nonetheless, may control the patients, the families, the nurses and health professionals generally. Their control may well be more powerful than any erudite oversimplification or its presentation.

Humanistic nusing practice theory in asking for phenomenological descriptions of the nurse's lived-world of experiencing proposes authentic awareness with the self of what is existent in the situation prior to conceptualization for dispersal. Unless nurses appreciate and give recognition to the dynamic meaningful breadth, depth, and future influence of their worlds the actualization of the potential thrust of the nursing professional will never be or become.

A THEORY OF NURSING

A human nurse nurses through a clinical process of "I-Thou, I-It, all-at-once to comfort."

"I-Thou" is a coming to know the other and the self in relation, intuitively. "I-It" is an authentic analyzing, synthesizing, and interpreting of the "I-Thou" relation through reflection.

The "all-at-once" symbolizes the multifarious multiplicities of extremes (incommensurables, criticals, nonconsequentials, contradictions, and inconsistencies) as metaphorically representative of what exists in the nurse's world.

"Comfort" is a state valued by a nurse as an aim in which a person is free to be and become, controlling and planning his own destiny, in accordance with his potential at a particular time in a particular situation.

APPENDIX

NURSE BEHAVIORS EXTRACTED
FROM CLINICAL DATA

In pursuing the idea of conceptualizing comfort as a proper aim of psychiatric nursing I extracted 12 nurse behaviors from my clinical data that were used repeatedly to increase patient comfort. I quantified these behaviors for two months. The following are a list of these behaviors with a representative example of all but the first. The first was too general and continuous for example.

1. I focused on recognizing patients by name, being certain I was correct about their names, and using their names often and appropriately. I also introduced myself. Names were viewed as supportive to the internalization of personal feelings of dignity and worth.

2. I interpreted, taught, and gave as much honest information as I could about patients' situations when it was sought or when puzzlement was apparent. This was based on the belief that it was their life, and choice was their prerogative since they were their own projects.

Examples

(a) While drinking coffee with a few patients at the dining room table suddenly we could hear Sidney, in his customary way, wailing, moaning, and muttering in another room. It is a sad sound. I was about to get up and go to him as I often do, when Arthur, who was sitting next to me, face working, and tense posture-wise, aggravatedly said, "Sidney doesn't have to do that, he should control himself, the rest of us control ourselves." I said, "When others express how miserable they feel, it sometimes arouses our own feelings about our misery." This was an attempt to provoke 32-year-old Arthur to work on his own

113

feelings of misery and to deter his projection of anger at himself out onto Sidney. Arthur looked at me sharply, like he had gotten the message, and agreed by relaxedly nodding his head.

(b)Alice, diagnosed as manic depressive, has been depressed. This depression dates from her going out to a department store and asking for a job. She was hired for a five-day-a-week job. This was done on her own. Later her readiness for a five-day-a-week job and her participation in the unit were questioned. Then Alice became depressed.

Alice was sitting in the dayroom. I sat down next to her. She looked very sad, her eyelids as well as her mouth, drooped. Her mouth worked as if she wanted to talk, but she was quiet. I asked her about her job decision. She said that she had not taken it. I said, "You look so sad that I feel like holding your hand." Her hands were in her coat pockets, but she looked at me and smiled weakly. I said, 'Sometimes a conflict of wanting to do two things at once in the present and not being able to can bring up the feelings of a past very much more important similar experience." Alice just shook her head up and down and looked at me. Alice is in her mid-forties. Later I was walking down the hall to leave saying goodbyes to various people. Alice came out of a side room, put both her hands out to me, and said, "goodbye and thank you." In a previous contact Alice had discussed her suicidal thoughts with me.

3. I verbalized my acceptance of patients' expressions of feelings with explanations of why I experienced these feelings of acceptance when I could do this authentically and appropriately.

Example

I met a new patient at coffee. Later she was the only patient in the dayroom when I went in. She had not spoken at coffee. Now she sat very stiffly in her chair. I sat down next to her and reintroduced myself. She looked scared but told me her name. Her shifting eyes reminded me of a cornered animal. She blurted out, "I don't believe I've met you." It was like she had said, "go away." I smiled at her and said, "We were introduced at coffee, but with so many new people it's hard to remember." Conversation continued to be tense. At one point Marion bolted from her chair toward the door. I thought she was going to leave. I stayed in my chair. She went to the fish bowl in the corner. We continued to talk about the fish. Marion came back and sat down a few seats away from me. I said that I felt I'd been asking her an awful lot of questions but that I was only trying to get to know her. Marion seemed to relax in her chair and gave a great deal of information about herself in a strange stiff sort of way often inserting a word that did not have meaning for me. I encouraged, supported and showed my interest . Finally she said that she had been admitted to McLean in her third year of nurses' training just before her psychiatric experience. She had been in therapy there, one-to-one for a couple of years. I teased her about knowing the ropes, yet giving me a difficult time. This was an attempt to increase her feelings of adequacy by bringing out the similarities of the old situation which she knew and this new situation. For the first time she really grinned at me, almost laughed. Marion is in her early thirties.

4. When verbalizations of acceptance were not appropriate, I acted out this acceptance by my behavior of staying with or doing for when appropriate.

Example

Mary is a middle-aged patient who, on her first days in the unit, was liberally gobbling her food with alertness for only more to be had. Her only rather loud, irrelevant, smiling expression was about her daughter who was a go-go dancer, had three children, and whom she had visited twice by bus in California. This day she approached me and asked if I would file her nails. I said that I would but asked if she know if there was a file in the unit. Another patient offered his. We sat down and I filed. The patient poured out a life story full of misery. This was a side of this patient that I had not perceived. I listened, nodded, and filed. The story started in the 1930s about her husband and mother-in-law's behavior; their marital separation; his being killed in World War II; their two children; their son, now thirty, was born with cerebral palsy, is blind and mute, and has been institutionalized since eleven months old; their daughter's husband left her with three children after fourteen years of marriage. I silently wondered what old feeling might have been aroused in her by her daughter's marital separation. Her daughter is so busy that she is unable to write regularly. She has told Mary not to worry if she doesn't hear from her. Mary then expressed concern over not receiving her usual letter this week from her mother, whom she visits. Mary had tried to reach her by phone and would again. I inquired if her mother lived alone. Yes, but next to relatives. She then related the drastic physical problems of a relative. I felt the sadness of this woman as she talked and empathized with the tough time she had had.

5. I expressed purposely, to burst assunder negative self concepts, my authentic human tender feelings for patients when appropriate and acceptable.

Example

I was sitting in a rather large group of patients in the dayroom. A casual conversation ensued about Thanksgiving as it had been and Christmas as it might be. There was talk of having been at home and plans for being at home. I supported and encouraged the discussion because of the meaningfulness of holidays, past and present. Snow was initiated as a topic. I said, "It would be nice to have a white Christmas, but not too white." Vincent, a stiff, exact, ritualistic person who avoids stepping in an obvious fashion on thresholds, does little jiggle-like dance steps before sitting down, and again before settling in his chair, suddenly spoke. "Josephine, I beg your pardon, but I must take issue with you." I encouraged his unusual behavioral expression. He went on and on about the importance of a white Christmas. I let my mind flow with his jumbled discourse trying to decipher what he was getting at rather than each specific rapidly mentioned issue. He went from white to black, day to night, goodness to badness, love to hate, this side of the world to the other side of the world (Vietnam). I expressed that he seemed to keep mentioning two sides of things and that for some reason I could not help thinking of boys and girls. I said that he was over on that side of the world (room) and that I was over on this side of the world. I asked why he did not come over to my side, paused a minute, felt this was asking too much of this patient, and said, "Well I'll come over to your side then." When I sat down next to Vincent, he giggled as he does. Arthur, a younger patient, made a critical jealous type comment about Vincent's age (50ish). Arthur has done this before when I give attention to Vincent. Has Arthur a stereotype of father images and perhaps mother images? I said to Vincent "you have beautiful white hair, and big, brown, smiling Italian eyes." Vincent sat back smiling shyly but comfortably and the discussion of the group continued.

6. I supported patients' rights to loving relationships with others: families, other staff, and other patients.

Example

Alice M. said that she was sad to be back at the hospital after her weekend at home. Alice is a quiet, bland, soft-spoken person about fifty. She wears a worried expression even when she smiles and strikes me like she is "turned inside" herself. I encourged her to talk about her time at home. She told me about how they had painted the living room with what for her was a show of real excitement. I said that her wish to be at home was very understandable. I did this because this patient almost whispers her wish to be at home and, generally, no one responds to it. Alice talked on with encouragement about the single sister whom she visits and the pleasure it gives her to be with this sister.
[I have other examples of this nurse behavior that indicate supporting of relationships between patients and between patients and other personnel.]

7. I showed respect for patients as persons with the rights to make as many choices for themselves as their current capabilities allowed.

Example

Discussion of group at coffee revolved around Carolyn's needing a new pair of shoes. The issues were where these might be gotten (Carolyn has money), what kind she should get, and who and when someone would take her for them. It struck me as if Carolyn might not have been present. I asked Carolyn what kind of shoes she would like. Carolyn responded that she did not know whether she should buy regular shoes, or sneakers, or canvas shoes like Marilyn had gotten. She beamed. Since, she has come up to me several times and discussed the two pairs of different kinds of shoes she bought and why. Carolyn is a sweet, simple, retarded, deaf sixty year old whose behavior resembles an eight year old.

8. I attempted to help patients consider their currently expressed feelings and behaviors in light of past life experiences and patterns, like and unlike their current ones.

Example

On my arrival after Christmas, Irene expressed anger at me in a laughing way for having been away. Then she moved from a seat in the corner of the room to a chair behind me at the coffee table. I moved to allow her to move up to the table, but she did not. After coffee Irene nonverbally with eyes and body movements told me to follow her. She led me into a small beauty parlor room and we both sat down. She closed her eyes. I said, "You seem to have some feelings about us all having been away." First she blurted, "I missed you," then in a quieter voice denied this, "It wasn't important that you weren't here." I said, "It could be helpful to you to talk about your present missing feelings as you had some very important losses of people when you were younger." Her eyes literally popped open and she again blurted, "You mean my parents?" I said, "Yes and your therapist could help you with this." I then asked if she ever had the opportunity to talk with anyone about such things. She replied, "No, well I had a social worker when I was a little girl." I tried at this point to transfer feelings of the past to the present. "Oh, for how long? What was she like?" "I don't remember," and Irene closed her eyes. In a few minutes Irene requested that I set her hair. She is capable of doing this herself. I set her hair, but discussed the question of what she was really asking for. I believe she was asking for concrete attention to test my ability to care for her. I was trying to say, concretely, by setting her hair, that people could care about her.

9. I encouraged patients' expression to come to understand better their behavioral messages to enable me to respond overtly as appropriately and therapeutically as possible.

Example

The previous time I was at the hospital Alice had not come to the unit. I was told that she felt too depressed to come down. I went to see her. She had looked surprised and impressed by my visit. She talked on at some length about her suicidal thoughts. I supported this on the basis that verbal expression might make active expression unnecessary if she experienced empathy regarding how dreadful she felt. Then with little encouragement she had come down to the unit with me. Today, Alice was always near me, but nonverbal except for concise responses to questions that were offered with effort. I verbalized my reflections on her behavior and said that I was wondering about it. She said, "I like having you around; it takes me away from my thoughts." "How are your thoughts?" "The same, I wonder if I'll ever get better?" "You've gotten better before. I wonder if you're not more concerned about whether you can stay well." Alice, eyes watery, agreed with a nod. Irene, another patient, interrupted, "Don't expect too much from me, I've been here twelve years." I responded to them both, "But, I do expect a lot of you; things don't always have to be the same."

10. I verified my intuitive grasp of how patients were experiencing events by questions and comments, and being alert to their responses.

Example

Vincent's ritualistic behavior is associated in my mind with his exaggerated conscious expression of only the true, the good, and the beautiful. On this occasion we had just had a long talk about his weekend at home, his concerns about his family, and his food likes and dislikes. As we left a room he took his usual long step over the threshold. I noted this aloud and asked him if he knew why he did this. His expression became wide-eyed and smiling which indicates to me he consciously or unconsciously is selecting what he is going to say. We came to the next threshold. He stopped me by touching my arm and said, "Josephine, I almost grabbed you to prevent your bumping into that patient." In relation to my last question I focused on the "grabbed you" and said, "Vincent, to think about grabbing me is a pretty natural thought, and no reason to take a wide step over a threshold." He put his foot very deliberately if rather testily, right in the middle of this threshold. He stopped, looked at me with his hands together and giggled. Then he had to go to the bathroom.

11. I attempted to encourage hope realistically through discussing individual therapeautic gains that could be derived from patients' investment in therapeutic opportunities available to them.

Example

My impression of Arthur, a thirty-two year old, is that he works at responding to me aggreeably as he thinks I want him to, he frequently goes out of his way to make cutting comments to me about middle-aged men patients, and he responds with anger or teasing to a female patient his age. Arthur has a mother, father, and two older sisters. He obviously let me win at Ping-pong several times. I discussed this with him and asked if he had ever talked with anyone about his responses to older women, people in general, or if he understood them. He said, "No, I have not been able to exactly figure this out yet." I repeated the talking it over. He said, "I haven't had much chance for that." Then staring at me he asked seriously, "Do you think talking it over would help?" I said, "I think that it would take a great deal of effort on your part, but I believe that it could help."

12. I supported appropriate patient self-images with as many concrete "hard to denies" as possible.

Example

Alice, a middle-aged woman, in the midst of a discussion of the difficulties of living outside the hospital, past relationships with nursing personnel, and her past practical nurse jobs suddenly said, "I worry about being sexually OK." This was kind of blurted out and she observed me closely. I said, "I thought that you had some concerns about this in relation to how you responded to my cutting the hairs on your face. I guess everyone worries at times about their adequacy in this area." She said, "I've never been able to have intercourse; I can just go as far as heavy petting. People say you can get a lot expressed if you have intercourse." I said, "Some people can, but if you have other standards that you've grown up with, (I suspect a rather religious, rigid Jewish background) it might cause difficulties to go against those standards." (Alice first became ill at sixteen, left school, and had some treatment in the community.) "It's pretty responsible not to be willing to bring a fatherless baby into the world, and I'm sure you'd have feelings about how your family might have responded to this sort of thing." Alice nodded and said "It's just that I don't know how womanly I am." I said with gestures and emphatically, "Well, Alice, if you have two things up here and no thing down here, then the fact is that you are a woman." Discussion pursued about her further talking about this topic with her therapist and the value of her working through her feelings in this area. This was a lengthy discussion and the first talking I had experienced Alice doing since her depression.

GLOSSARY

angular view.   An individual's unique vision of reality necessarily restricted by the angle of his particular here and now.

authenticity.   Genuineness; congruence with the self.

(the) between.   The realm of the intersubjective.

bracket.   Hold in abeyance.

community.   Two or more persons struggling together toward a center.

existential.   Of, relating to, or affirming existence; grounded in existence or the experience of living.

existential dialogue.   A unique individual person with the wholeness of his being is present, open to, and relates to the other seen in his unique individual wholeness; an exchange in which two persons transcend themselves and participate in the other's being; an interior unification; a mutual common union in being.

existential experience.   Contact with reality with the whole of one's being; involves all that a man *is* as opposed to experiencing through one or several faculties.

existentialism.   Philosophy based on phenomenological studies of reality; centers on the analysis of existence particularly of the individual human being, stresses the freedom and responsibility of the individual, regards human existence as not completely describable or understandable in idealistic or scientific terms.

here and now.   An individual's unique experience of his present spatial and temporal reality including his past experiences and expectations of the future.

humanistic nursing.   A theory and practice that rest on an existential philosophy, value experiencing and the evolving of the "new," and aim at phenomenological description of the art-science of nursing viewed as a lived intersubjective transactional experience; nursing seen within its human context.

intersubjective.   Pertaining to two or mure human persons and their shared between; a relationship of two or more human beings in which each is the originator of human acts and responses.

121

lived dialogue. A form of existential intersubjective relating expressed in being with and doing with the other who is regarded as a presence (as opposed to an object); a lived call and response.

lived world. The everyday world as it is experienced in the here and now.

metanursing. A discipline designed to deal critically with nursing, ontological study of nursing; study of the phenomenon of nursing; a critical study of nursing within its human context.

metatheoretical. Transcending theory; ontological inquiry from which theory may be derived.

nursology. Study of the phenomenon of nursing aimed toward the development of nursing theory.

phenomenology. The descriptive study of phenomena.

phenomenon. An observable fact, event, occurrence or circumstance; an appearance or immediate object of awareness in experience. A phenomenon may be objective (that is, external to the person aware of it) or subjective (for example, a thought or feeling).

prereflective experience. Primary awareness or perception of reality not yet thought about; spontaneous experience; immediate experience or perception.

presence. A mode of being available or open in a situation with the wholeness of one's unique individual being; a gift of the self which can only be given freely, invoked, or evoked.

transactional. An aware knowing of one's effect in a situation of which one is a part; an action that goes both ways between persons.

SELECTED BIBLIOGRAPHY

In addition to the extensive discussions that have been generated since the initial publication of Paterson and Zderad's *Humanistic Hursing,* the work has been formally cited and or discussed in the nursing literature. This selected bibliography was compiled by Helen Streubert, MSN, RN doctoral candidate and research assistant in the Department of Nursing Education, Teachers College/Columbia University, New York.

BOOKS

Chenitz, W.C. (1986). *From practice to grounded theory.* Menlo Park, California: Addison-Wesley.

Chinn, P.O., & Jacobs, M.K. (1983). *Theory and nursing.* St. Louis: Mosby Company.

Duldt, B.W. (1985). *Theoretical perspectives for nursing.* Boston: Little-Brown & Company

Ellis, R. (1984). Philosophic inquiry. In H.H. Werley & J.J. Fitzpatrick (Eds.), *Annual review of nursing research* (pp. 211-228). New York: Springer Publishing Company.

Fitzpatrick, J., & Whall, A. (1983). *Conceptual models of nursing: Analysis application.* Bowie, Maryland: Brady Company

Kleiman, S. (1986). Humanistic nursing: The phenomenological theory of Paterson and Zderad. In P. Winstead-Fry (Ed.), *Case studies in nursing theory* (pp. 167-195). New York: National League for Nursing.

Leininger, M. (1985). Ethnography and ethnonursing models and modes of qualitative data analysis. In M. Leininger (Ed.), *Qualitative research methods in nursing.* Orlando, Florida: Grune & Stratton.

Meleis, A.I. (1985). Theoretical nursing: Development and progress. Philadelphia: Lippincott.

Moccia, P. (Ed.). (1986). *New approaches to theory development.* New York: National League for Nursing.

Munhall, P.L., & Oiler, C.J. (1986), *Nursing research: A qualitative perspective.* Norwalk, Connecticut: Appleton-Century-Crofts.

Paterson, J.G. (1978). The tortuous way toward nursing theory. In *Theory development: What, why, how?* (pp. 49-65). New York: National League for Nursing.

Phipps, W.J., Long, B.C., & Woods, N.F. (1987). *Medical – surgical nursing: Concepts and clinical practice* (3rd ed.). St. Louis: Mosby Company.

Roy, C. (1984). *Introduction to nursing: An adaptation model* (2nd ed.). Englewood Cliffs, NJ: Prentice–Hall, Inc.

Stevens, B.J. (1984). *Nursing theory: Analysis, application, evaluation* (2nd ed.). Boston: Little Brown Co.

Suppe, F., & Jacox, A. (1985). Philosophy of science and the development of nursing theory. In H.H. Werley &J.J. Fitzpatrick (Eds.), *Annual review of nursing research* (pp. 241-267). New York: Springer Publishing Company.

Zderad, L.T. (1978). From here-and-now to theory: Refelections on "how". In *Theory development: What, why, how (pp. 35-48). New York: National League for Nursing.*

ARTICLES

Bael, E.D., & Lowry, B.J. (1987). Patient and situational factors that affect nursing students' like or dislike of caring for patient. *Nursing Research, 36* (5), 298-302.

Beckstrand, J. (1980). A critique of several conceptions of practice theory in nursing. *Research in Nursing and Health, 3,* 69-79.

Bottorff, J.L., & Dcruz, J.V. (1984). Towards inclusive notions of patient and nurse. *Journal of Advanced Nursing, 9* (6), 549-553.

Braun J.L., Baines, S.L., Olson, N.G., & Scruby, L.S. (1984). *Health Values, 8* (3), 12-15.

Brown, L. (1986). The experience of care: Patient perspectives. *Topics in Clinical Nursing, 8* (2), 56-62.

Chenitz, W.C., & Swanson, J.M. (1984). Surfacing nursing process—A method for generating nursing theory from practice. *Journal of Advanced Nursing, 9* (2), 205-215.

Drew, N. (1986). Exclusion and confirmation: A phenomenology of patients' experiences with caregivers. *Image, 18* (2), 39-43.

Flaskerud, J.H. (1986). On toward a theory of nursing action skills and competency in nurse-patient interaction. *Nursing Research, 35* (4), 250-252.

King, E.C. (1984). Humanistic education: Theory and teaching strategies. *Nurse Education 8 (4), 39 – 42.*

Nahon, N.E. (1982). The relationship of self-disclosure, interpersonal dependency, and life changes to loneliness in young adults. *Nursing Research, 31* (6), 343-347.

Oiler, C. (1982). The phenomenological approach in nursing research. *Nursing Research, 31* (3) 178-181.

Rigdon, I.S., Clayton, B.C., & Dimond, M. (1987). Toward a theory of helpfulness for the elderly bereaved: An invitation to a new life. *Advances in Nursing Science, 9* (2), 32-43.

Sarter, B. (1987). Evolutionary idealism: A philosophical foundation for holistic nursing theory. *Advances in Nursing Science, 9* (2), 1-9.

Taylor, S.G. (1985). Rights and responsibilities: Nurse patient relationships. *Image, 17* (1), 9-16.

INDEX

Socrates, 38
Space, 18–20, 34–35
Subjective-objective, 27, 35–36, 52, 67, 79, 81, 93
Synthesis, 72–74, 79, 82–84, 93, 95, 102, 103, 108, 111. *See also* Complementary synthesis

Theory, *see* Humanistic nursing practice theory
Time, 18–20, 29, 33–34
Transactions, 11, 12–13, 16–20, 21, 35–36. *See also* Between, (the); Dialogue; Intersubjective; and Presence
Trautman, Mary Jane, 87, 88

Uniqueness, 4, 7, 15, 23, 25, 26, 27, 32, 34, 35–36, 40, 45, 56, 68, 69, 72, 77, 111

Value, 6, 16, 17, 18, 30, 39, 46–48, 54, 56–57, 69, 71, 77, 79, 85, 97, 98, 104, 105

Well-being, 12, 16, 36, 89, 92
Whitehead, Alfred North, 6
Wiesel, Elie, 7, 96
Weymouth, Lilyan, 55
Words, 8, 60–62, 73, 81, 98
Wright, Edward A., 91